ACADEMIC SKILLS
PROBLEMS WORKBOOK

The Guilford School Practitioner Series

EDITORS

STEPHEN N. ELLIOTT, PhD
Vanderbilt University

JOSEPH C. WITT, PhD
Louisiana State University, Baton Rouge

Recent Volumes

Academic Skills Problems Workbook, Revised Edition
Edward S. Shapiro

Academic Skills Problems: Direct Assessment and Intervention, Third Edition
Edward S. Shapiro

ADHD in the Schools, Second Edition: Assessment and Intervention Strategies
George J. DuPaul and Gary Stoner

Helping Schoolchildren Cope with Anger: A Cognitive-Behavioral Intervention
Jim Larson and John E. Lochman

Child Abuse and Neglect: The School's Response
Connie Burrows Horton and Tracy K. Cruise

Traumatic Brain Injury in Children and Adolescents: Assessment and Intervention
Margaret Semrud-Clikeman

Schools and Families: Creating Essential Connections for Learning
Sandra L. Christenson and Susan M. Sheridan

Homework Success for Children with ADHD:
A Family–School Intervention Program
Thomas J. Power, James L. Karustis, and Dina F. Habboushe

Conducting School-Based Assessments of Child and Adolescent Behavior
Edward S. Shapiro and Thomas R. Kratochwill, Editors

Designing Preschool Interventions: A Practitioner's Guide
David W. Barnett, Susan H. Bell, and Karen T. Carey

Effective School Interventions
Natalie Rathvon

DSM-IV Diagnosis in the Schools
Alvin E. House

Medications for School-Age Children: Effects on Learning and Behavior
Ronald T. Brown and Michael G. Sawyer

Advanced Applications of Curriculum-Based Measurement
Mark R. Shinn, Editor

Academic Skills
Problems Workbook

Revised Edition

◆ ◆ ◆

Edward S. Shapiro

◆

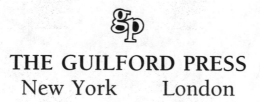

THE GUILFORD PRESS
New York   London

© 2004 The Guilford Press
A Division of Guilford Publications, Inc.
72 Spring Street, New York, NY 10012
www.guilford.com

Printed in the United States of America

This book is printed on acid-free paper.

Last digit is print number: 9 8 7 6 5 4 3 2 1

ISBN 1-57230-968-7

◆ ◆ ◆
About the Author
◆

Edward S. Shapiro, PhD, is Iacocca Professor of Education, Professor of School Psychology, and Director of the Center for Promoting Research to Practice at Lehigh University, Lehigh, Pennsylvania. He is also Executive Director of Lehigh Transition and Assessment Services, which provides training in the school-to-work transition for secondary school-age students and young adults with disabilities. A recipient of the Lightner Witmer Award from the Division of School Psychology of the American Psychological Association, in recognition of early career contributions to school psychology, he is past Editor of *School Psychology Review,* the official journal of the National Association of School Psychologists. Dr. Shapiro has written numerous books and publications in the areas of curriculum-based assessment, behavioral assessment, behavioral interventions, and self-management strategies for classroom behavior change, including *Conducting School-Based Assessments of Child and Adolescent Behavior* and *Behavioral Assessment in Schools, Second Edition: Theory, Research, and Clinical Foundations* (both coedited with Thomas R. Kratochwill), and *Promoting Children's Health: Integrating School, Family, and Community* (coauthored with Thomas J. Power, George J. DuPaul, and Anne E. Kazak). He is currently codirecting a federal training project focused on developing doctoral school psychologists as pediatric school psychologists, a model of training that attempts to train students to integrate health, psychological, and educational needs for children within school settings.

Contents

STEP 2. ASSESSING INSTRUCTIONAL PLACEMENT

STEP 3. INSTRUCTIONAL MODIFICATION

STEP 4. PROGRESS MONITORING

List of Forms

ACADEMIC SKILLS
PROBLEMS WORKBOOK

♦♦♦
Introduction
♦

The purpose of this workbook is to provide forms, instructions, and other materials to supplement *Academic Skills Problems: Direct Assessment and Intervention* (3rd edition). The workbook offers elaboration and detail of material covered in the text, and also provides additional forms to supplement those in the text. Some forms in the text are duplicated in the workbook for ease in copying; users of the manual are granted permission from the publisher to copy and modify these forms for their personal use. Although the workbook can certainly be used on its own, its purpose is to complement rather than stand independent from the text.

The workbook also offers opportunities for learning, practicing, and mastering many of the skills discussed in the text. For example, a complete manual related to use of the Behavioral Observation of Students in Schools (BOSS) observation code is provided. In addition, information is provided on using the BOSS software (available from The Psychological Corporation®; *www.harcourtassessment.com*) designed to use as an alternative of the BOSS paper-and-pencil version. Full definitions of the BOSS behavioral categories, as well as instructions for collecting information, scoring the observations, and interpreting the data, are given. Also included are forms for completing teacher and student interviews, along with a useful checklist for obtaining teacher reports for academic behavior.

In the area of conducting the direct assessment of academic skills, the workbook offers additional instructions and practice exercises in how these procedures are used. In particular, detailed explanations of using such measures as "digits correct per minute" and "correct letter sequences" to score math and spelling, respectively, are provided. The workbook also offers a description of and exercises in how to graph data, collect local norms, and other tasks related to a direct assessment of academic skills.

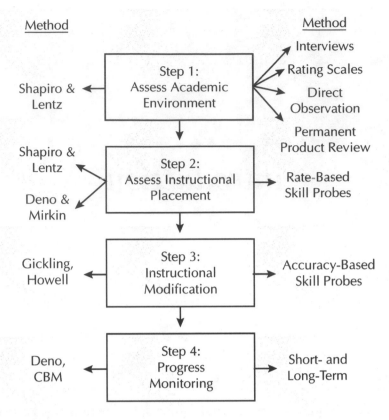

FIGURE 1. Model of direct assessment of academic skills. Adapted from Shapiro (1991, p. 331). Copyright 1990 by the National Association of School Psychologists. Adapted by permission of the author.

The workbook follows the model of assessment described in the *Academic Skills Problems* text and depicted in Figure 1. The first section, corresponding to the first step of the assessment process—assessing the academic environment (see Figure 2)—provides materials for interviewing teachers and students, conducting direct observations, and using informant report data (teacher rating scale). The next section, corresponding to Step 2 of the process—assessing instructional placement—provides information related to the processes involved in direct assessment of academic skills (in particular, details about the assessment of reading, math, spelling, and written language). This section contains information on both the use of short- and long-term data collection procedures.

The third section of the workbook offers details on the use of a powerful instructional intervention: the "folding-in" technique. The final section, corresponding to Step 4 of the model—progress monitoring—provides important information about the graphic display of data, as well as how to collect local norms.

Throughout, the reader will find detailed "how to" explanations offered in a step-by-step fashion. Practice exercises are also provided, and readers are encouraged to develop their own exercises modeled on those in the workbook.

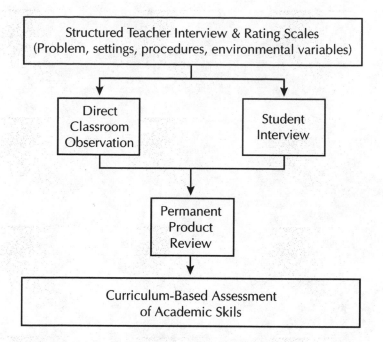

FIGURE 2. Sequences of methods in conducting Steps 1 and 2 of the direct assessment of academic skills.

STEP 1

♦♦♦

Assessing the Academic Environment

♦

♦♦♦
Teacher Interview
♦

The assessment process begins with the teacher interview. Several forms are provided to facilitate the interview. The first, which is also printed in the text, suggests the specific questions that should be addressed for each academic area when interviewing teachers. Designed primarily to be completed during a face-to-face meeting with a teacher, the form can also be given to the teacher to fill out before the interview actually occurs. When the form is used in this way, the information provided by the teacher can be used as the context for more in-depth discussion. In the interview process, it is important to learn from the teacher the nature of interventions that have already been tried or are currently in place. In addition, obtaining an understanding of the "big picture" of skill development in reading and mathematics is a critical part of fully understanding the student's problem from the teacher's perspective. In reading, assessing a student's knowledge base in phonemic awareness, alphabetic principle, vocabulary, fluency, and comprehension is essential. In mathematics, information on a student's acquisition of computational skills and concepts–applications of mathematical principles is needed. These components are embedded in the interview form.

Form 1

TEACHER INTERVIEW FORM FOR ACADEMIC PROBLEMS

Student: _____   Teacher: _____

Birth date: _____   Date: _____

Grade: _____   School: _____

                                Interviewer: _____

GENERAL

Why was this student referred? _____

_____

What type of academic problem(s) does this student have?

_____

READING

Primary type of reading series used   Secondary type of reading materials used

☐ Basal reader   ☐ Basal reader

☐ Literature-based   ☐ Literature-based

☐ Trade books   ☐ Trade books

                                             ☐ None

Reading series title (if applicable) _____

   Grade level of series currently placed _____

   Title of book in series currently placed _____

How many groups do you teach? _____

Which group is this student assigned to? _____

At this point in the school year, where is the average student in your class reading?

   Level and book _____

   Place in book (beg., mid., end, specific page) _____

   Time allotted/day for reading _____

How is time divided? (Independent seatwork? Small group? Cooperative groups? Large groups?)

_____

_____

How is placement in reading program determined? _____

_____

How are changes made in the program? _____

_____

Does this student participate in remedial reading programs? How much?

_____

Typical daily instructional procedures _____

_____

Contingencies for accuracy? _____

_____

Contingencies for completion? _____

_____

Types of interventions already attempted:

    Simple (e.g., reminders, cues, self-monitoring, motivation, feedback, instructions):

_____

_____

    Moderate (e.g., increasing time of existing instruction, extra tutoring sessions):

_____

_____

    Intensive (e.g., changed curriculum, changed instructional modality,
    changed instructional grouping, added intensive one-to-one):

_____

_____

Frequency and duration of interventions used:

_____

_____

Extent to which interventions were successful:

_____

_____

Daily scores (if available) for past 2 weeks _____

_____

Group standardized test results (if available) _____

_____

ORAL READING

How does he/she read orally compared to others in his/her reading group?

____ Much worse   ____ Somewhat worse   ____ About the same

____ Somewhat better   ____ Much better

In the class?

____ Much worse   ____ Somewhat worse   ____ About the same

____ Somewhat better   ____ Much better

WORD ATTACK

Does he/she attempt unknown words? _____

WORD KNOWLEDGE/SIGHT VOCABULARY

How does the student's word knowledge (vocabulary) compare to others in his/her reading group?

____ Much worse   ____ Somewhat worse   ____ About the same

____ Somewhat better   ____ Much better

In the class?

____ Much worse   ____ Somewhat worse   ____ About the same

____ Somewhat better   ____ Much better

How does the student's sight-word vocabulary compare to others in his/her reading group?

____ Much worse   ____ Somewhat worse   ____ About the same

____ Somewhat better   ____ Much better

In the class?

____ Much worse   ____ Somewhat worse   ____ About the same

____ Somewhat better   ____ Much better

COMPREHENSION

How well does the student seem to understand what he/she reads compared to others in his/her reading group?

_____ Much worse   _____ Somewhat worse   _____ About the same

_____ Somewhat better   _____ Much better

In the class?

_____ Much worse   _____ Somewhat worse   _____ About the same

_____ Somewhat better   _____ Much better

Areas of comprehension where student has success (+)/difficulty (–):

_____ Main ideas

_____ Prediction

_____ Recollection of facts

_____ Identifying plot

_____ Identifying main characters

_____ Synthesizing the story

_____ Other (describe):

_____

_____

BEHAVIOR DURING READING

Rate the following areas from 1 to 5 (1 = very unsatisfactory, 3 = satisfactory, 5 = superior).

Reading Group

a. Oral reading ability (as evidenced in reading group)   _____
b. Volunteers answers   _____
c. When called upon, gives correct answer   _____
d. Attends to other students when they read aloud   _____
e. Knows the appropriate place in book   _____

Independent Seatwork

a. Stays on task   _____
b. Completes assigned work in required time   _____
c. Work is accurate   _____
d. Works quietly   _____
e. Remains in seat when required   _____

Homework (if any)

a. Handed in on time ____
b. Is complete ____
c. Is accurate ____

MATHEMATICS

Curriculum series _____

What are the specific problems in math? _____

_____

Time allotted/day for math _____

How is time divided? (Independent seatwork? Small group? Large group?
Cooperative groups?) _____

_____

Are your students grouped in math? _____

If so, how many groups do you have, and in which group is this student placed? _____

_____

For an **average** performing student in your class, at what point in the planned course
format would you consider this student at mastery?

   (See computational mastery form.) _____

_____

For an **average** performing student in your class, at what point in the planned course
format would you consider this student instructional?

   (See computational mastery form.) _____

_____

For an **average** performing student in your class, at what point in the planned course
format would you consider this student frustrational?

   (See computational mastery form.) _____

_____

For the **targeted** student in your class, at what point in the planned course format would
you consider this student at mastery?

   (See computational mastery form.) _____

_____

For the **targeted** student in your class, at what point in the planned course format would you consider this student instructional?

    (See computational mastery form.) _____

_____

For the **targeted** student in your class, at what point in the planned course format would you consider this student frustrational?

    (See computational mastery form.) _____

_____

How is mastery assessed? _____

Describe any difficulties this student has in applying math skills in these areas:

    Numeration _____

    Estimation _____

    Time _____

    Money _____

    Measurement _____

    Geometry _____

    Graphic display _____

    Interpretation of graph _____

    Word problems _____

    Other _____

How are changes made in the student's math program? _____

_____

Does this student participate in remedial math programs? _____

Typical daily instructional procedures _____

_____

_____

Contingencies for accuracy? _____

_____

Contingencies for completion? _____

_____

Types of interventions already attempted:

Simple (e.g., reminders, cues, self-monitoring, motivation, feedback, instructions):

_____

_____

Moderate (e.g., increasing time of existing instruction, extra tutoring sessions):

_____

_____

Intensive (e.g., changed curriculum, changed instructional modality,
changed instructional grouping, added intensive one-to-one):

_____

_____

Frequency and duration of interventions used:

_____

_____

Extent to which interventions were successful:

_____

_____

Daily scores (if available) for past 2 weeks _____

_____

Group standardized test results (if available) _____

_____

BEHAVIOR DURING MATH

Rate the following areas from 1 to 5 (1 = very unsatisfactory, 3 = satisfactory, 5 = superior)

Math Group (large)

a. Volunteers answers _____
b. When called upon, gives correct answer _____
c. Attends to other students when they give answers _____
d. Knows the appropriate place in math book _____

Math Group (small)

a. Volunteers answers
b. When called upon, gives correct answer ____
c. Attends to other students when they give answers ____
d. Knows the appropriate place in math book ____

Math Group (cooperative)

a. Volunteers answers
b. Contributes to group objectives ____
c. Attends to other students when they give answers ____
d. Facilitates others in group to participate ____
e. Shows appropriate social skills in group ____

Independent Seatwork

a. Stays on task
b. Completes assigned work in required time ____
c. Work is accurate ____
d. Works from initial directions ____
e. Works quietly ____
f. Remains in seat when required ____

Homework (if any)

a. Handed in on time
b. Is complete ____
c. Is accurate ____

SPELLING

Type of material used for spelling instruction:
    ☐ Published spelling series

        Title of series _____

    ☐ Basal reading series

        Title of series _____

    ☐ Teacher-made materials _____

    ☐ Other _____

Level of instruction (if applicable) _____

At this point in the school year, where is the average student in your class spelling?
    Level, place in book _____

Time allotted/day for spelling _____

How is time divided? (Independent seatwork? Small group? Cooperative groups?)

_____

_____

How is placement in the spelling program determined? _____

_____

How are changes made in the program? _____

_____

Typical daily instructional procedures _____

_____

Types of interventions already attempted:

Simple (e.g., reminders, cues, self-monitoring, motivation, feedback, instructions):

_____

_____

Moderate (e.g., increasing time of existing instruction, extra tutoring sessions):

_____

_____

Intensive (e.g., changed curriculum, changed instructional modality,
changed instructional grouping, added intensive one-to-one):

_____

_____

Frequency and duration of interventions used:

_____

_____

Extent to which interventions were successful:

_____

_____

Contingencies for accuracy? _____

_____

Contingencies for completion? _____

_____

WRITING

Please describe the type of writing assignments you give? _____

_____

Compared to others in your class, does he/she have difficulty with (please provide brief descriptions):

☐ Expressing thoughts _____

☐ Story length _____

☐ Story depth _____

☐ Creativity _____

Mechanics:

☐ Capitalization

☐ Punctuation

☐ Grammar

☐ Handwriting

☐ Spelling

Comments: _____

_____

BEHAVIOR

Are there social–behavioral adjustment problems interfering with this student's academic progress? (be specific)

_____

_____

Check any item that describes this student's behavior:

_____ Distracted, short attention span, unable to concentrate

_____ Hyperactive, constant, aimless movement

_____ Impulsive aggressive behaviors, lacks self-control

_____ Fluctuating levels of performance

_____ Frequent negative self-statements

_____ Unconsciously repeating verbal or motor acts

_____ Lethargic, sluggish, too quiet

_____ Difficulty sharing or working with others

ELEMENTARY MATH WHOLE-NUMBER COMPUTATIONAL
SKILLS MASTERY CURRICULUM

GRADE 1

1. Add two one-digit numbers: sums to 10
2. Subtract two one-digit numbers: combinations to 10

GRADE 2

3. Add two one-digit numbers: sums 11–19
4. Add a one-digit number to a two-digit number—no regrouping
5. Add a two-digit number to a two-digit number—no regrouping
6. Add a three-digit number to a three-digit number—no regrouping
7. Subtract a one-digit number from a one- or two-digit number—combinations to 18
8. Subtract a one-digit number from a two-digit number—no regrouping
9. Subtract a two-digit number from a two-digit number—no regrouping
10. Subtract a three-digit number from a three-digit number—no regrouping
11. Multiplication facts—0's, 1's, 2's

GRADE 3

12. Add three or more one-digit numbers
13. Add three or more two-digit numbers—no regrouping
14. Add three or more three- and four-digit numbers—no regrouping
15. Add a one-digit number to a two-digit number with regrouping
16. Add a two-digit number to a two-digit number with regrouping
17. Add a two-digit number to a three-digit number with regrouping from the 10's column only
18. Add a two-digit number to a three-digit number with regrouping from the 100's column only
19. Add a two-digit number to a three-digit number with regrouping from 10's and 100's columns
20. Add a three-digit number to a three-digit number with regrouping from the 10's column only
21. Add a three-digit number to a three-digit number with regrouping from the 100's column only
22. Add a three-digit number to a three-digit number with regrouping from the 10's and 100's columns
23. Add a four-digit number to a four-digit number with regrouping in one to three columns
24. Subtract two four-digit numbers—no regrouping
25. Subtract a one-digit number from a two-digit number with regrouping
26. Subtract a two-digit number from a two-digit number with regrouping

27. Subtract a two-digit number from a three-digit number with regrouping from the 10's column only
28. Subtract a two-digit number from a three-digit number with regrouping from the 100's column only
29. Subtract a two-digit number from a three-digit number with regrouping from the 10's and 100's columns
30. Subtract a three-digit number from a three-digit number with regrouping from the 10's column only
31. Subtract a three-digit number from a three-digit number with regrouping from the 100's column only
32. Subtract a three-digit number from a three-digit number with regrouping from the 10's and 100's columns
33. Multiplication facts—3–9

GRADE 4

34. Add a five- or six-digit number to a five- or six-digit number with regrouping in any columns
35. Add three or more two-digit numbers with regrouping
36. Add three or more three-digit numbers with regrouping
37. Subtract a five- or six-digit number from a five- or six-digit number with regrouping in any columns
38. Multiply a two-digit number by a one-digit number with no regrouping
39. Multiply a three-digit number by a one-digit number with no regrouping
40. Multiply a two-digit number by a one-digit number with no regrouping
41. Multiply a three-digit number by a one-digit number with regrouping
42. Division facts—0–9
43. Divide a two-digit number by a one-digit number with no remainder
44. Divide a two-digit number by a one-digit number with remainder
45. Divide a three-digit number by a one-digit number with remainder
46. Divide a four-digit number by a one-digit number with remainder

GRADE 5

47. Multiply a two-digit number by a two-digit number with regrouping
48. Multiply a three-digit number by a two-digit number with regrouping
49. Multiply a three-digit number by a three-digit number with regrouping

Interviews with teachers should be guided by the need to obtain general information about how a teacher manages instruction, the classroom environment, and the nature of strategies already attempted to remediate the problem behavior of the student. Included in the interview is information about the success or failure of these strategies. In addition or instead of using a semistructured interviewing form, some evaluators may prefer to be guided by more general questions. This format specifically asks questions around instructional practices, curriculum, assessment, and management. Typically, the interview is conducted following an observation of the teacher teaching the student of interest. The following questions are useful to guide this type of interview process.

QUESTIONS TO GUIDE GENERAL TEACHER INTERVIEWS
FOR ACADEMIC SKILLS*

Teacher _____   Student _____

Academic subject(s) _____   Date _____

1. What was the specific instructional assignment being taught during the observation?

2. How was the instructional assignment presented to the student?

3. What opportunities were presented for guided practice?

4. What opportunities were presented for independent practice?

5. What opportunities were presented for feedback to students?

6. What were the specific objectives of the instructional lesson observed?

7. How did you determine whether the student was successful during the lesson observed?

8. What type of additional support beyond your normal classroom instruction does this student need to succeed?

9. What strategies seem to work with this student?

10. What strategies do not seem to work with this student?

11. What types of assessment information do you collect?

12. How do you use the information gathered about student performance?

13. During group instruction, what clues do you use to evaluate a student's performance?

14. What adaptations do you make or permit of assignments?

15. What adaptations do you make or permit on tests?

16. What kind of support can you expect from supervisors and administrators for more intensive intervention changes that are needed?

*Many thanks to Christine Schubel, EdS, for her contributions to this form.

◆◆◆
Academic Performance Rating Scale
◆

Another approach to gathering information about student academic performance and classroom structure is to use a teacher rating scale. DuPaul, Rapport, and Perriello (1991) developed the Academic Performance Rating Scale designed to provide teacher-based ratings of student performance in math and language arts among students in grades 1 through 6. The factor analysis of the scale results in three subscales: Academic Success, Impulse Control, and Academic Productivity (as judged by the teacher) (see Table 1). Normative data divided by gender along with instructions for scoring for each factor ,are provided (see Table 2).

Note that items 12, 13, 15, 16, 17, 18, and 19 are reversed scored (i.e., 5 = 1; 4 = 2; 3 = 3; 2 = 4; 1 = 5), so that the total higher scores always reflect more desirable outcomes.

Form 4

ACADEMIC PERFORMANCE RATING SCALE*

Student _____   Date _____

Age _____   Grade _____   Teacher _____

For each of the items below, please estimate the above student's performance over the PAST WEEK. For each item, please circle one choice only.

1. Estimate the percentage of written **math work** completed (regardless of accuracy) relative to classmates.	0–49% 1	50–69% 2	70–79% 3	80–89% 4	90–100% 5
2. Estimate the percentage of written **language arts** work completed (regardless of accuracy) relative to classmates.	0–49% 1	50–69% 2	70–79% 3	80–89% 4	90–100% 5
3. Estimate the accuracy of completed written **math** work (i.e., percent correct of work done).	0–64% 1	65–69% 2	70–79% 3	80–89% 4	90–100% 5
4. Estimate the accuracy of completed written **language arts** work (i.e., percent correct of work done).	0–64% 1	65–69% 2	70–79% 3	80–89% 4	90–100% 5
5. How consistent has the quality of this child's academic work been over the past week?	Consistently poor 1	More poor than successful 2	Variable 3	More successful than poor 4	Consistently successful 5
6. How frequently does the student accurately follow teacher instructions and/or class discussion during *large-group* (e.g., whole class) instruction?	Never 1	Rarely 2	Sometimes 3	Often 4	Very often 5
7. How frequently does the student accurately follow teacher instructions and/or class discussion during *small-group* (e.g., reading group) instruction?	Never 1	Rarely 2	Sometimes 3	Often 4	Very often 5
8. How quickly does the child learn new material (i.e., pick up novel concepts)?	Very slowly 1	Slowly 2	Average 3	Quickly 4	Very quickly 5

9. What is the quality or neatness of this child's handwriting?	Poor	Fair	Average	Above average	Excellent
	1	2	3	4	5
10. What is the quality of this child's reading skills?	Poor	Fair	Average	Above average	Excellent
	1	2	3	4	5
11. What is the quality of this child'is writing skills?	Poor	Fair	Average	Above average	Excellent
	1	2	3	4	5
12. How often does the child complete written work in a careless, hasty fashion?	Never 5	Rarely 4	Sometimes 3	Often 2	Very often 1
13. How frequently does the child take more time to complete work than his/her classmates?	Never 5	Rarely 4	Sometimes 3	Often 2	Very often 1
14. How often is the child able to pay attention without you prompting him/her?	Never 5	Rarely 4	Sometimes 3	Often 2	Very often 1
15. How frequently does this child require your assistance to accurately complete his/her academic work?	Never 5	Rarely 4	Sometimes 3	Often 2	Very often 1
16. How often does the child begin written work prior to understanding the directions?	Never 5	Rarely 4	Sometimes 3	Often 2	Very often 1
17. How frequently does this child have difficulty recalling material from a previous day's lessons?	Never 5	Rarely 4	Sometimes 3	Often 2	Very often 1
18. How often does the child appear to be staring excessively or "spaced out"?	Never 5	Rarely 4	Sometimes 3	Often 2	Very often 1
19. How often does the child appear withdrawn or tend to lack an emotional response in a social situation?	Never 5	Rarely 4	Sometimes 3	Often 2	Very often 1

*From DuPaul, Rapport, and Perriello (1991, pp. 299–300). Copyright 1991 by the National Association of School Psychologists. Reprinted by permission.

APRS SCORING INSTRUCTIONS:

Step 1: Write in the score assigned by the teacher for each item in the blank column.

Step 2: Sum the columns and write the total in the last row.

Item #	Academic Success	Impulse Control	Academic Productivity
1			
2			
3			
4			
5			
6			
7			
8			
9			
10			
11			
12**			
13**			
14			
15**			
16**			
17**			
18**			
19**			
TOTALS	Academic Success score	Impulse Control score	Academic Productivity score

**These items have been reversed scored.

26

TABLE 1. Factor Structure of the Academic Performance Rating Scale (APRS)

Scale item	Academic Success	Impulse Control	Academic Productivity
1. Math work completed	.30	−.02	**.84**
2. Language arts completed	.32	.06	**.82**
3. Math work accuracy	**.68**	.17	.50
4. Language arts accuracy	**.68**	.17	.50
5. Consistency of work	.50	.21	**.72**
6. Follows group instructions	.41	.35	**.69**
7. Follows small-group instructions	.39	.37	**.64**
8. Learns material quickly	**.81**	.17	.39
9. Neatness of handwriting	.41	**.50**	.31
10. Quality of reading	**.87**	.16	.23
11. Quality of speaking	**.80**	.20	.21
12. Careless work completion	.15	**.72**	.36
13. Time to complete work	.36	.21	**.61**
14. Attention without prompts	.24	.35	**.53**
15. Requires assistance	.44	.39	**.53**
16. Begins work carelessly	.16	**.82**	.02
17. Recall difficulties	**.66**	.35	.38
18. Stare excessively	.19	.39	**.67**
19. Social withdrawal	.16	.28	**.57**
Estimate of % variance	55.5	6.6	6.1

Note. Boldface values indicate items included in the factor named in the column head. From DuPaul, Rapport, and Perriello (1991, p. 290). Copyright 1991 by the National Association of School Psychologists. Reprinted by permission.

TABLE 2. Means and Standard Deviation for the APRS by Grade and Gender

Grade	Total score	Academic Success	Impulse Control	Academic Productivity
Grade 1 (*n* = 82)				
Girls (*n* = 40)	67.02 (16.27)	23.92 (7.37)	9.76 (2.49)	44.68 (10.91)
Boys (*n* = 42)	71.95 (16.09)	26.86 (6.18)	10.67 (2.82)	46.48 (11.24)
Grade 2 (*n* = 91)				
Girls (*n* = 46)	72.56 (12.33)	26.61 (5.55)	10.15 (2.70)	47.85 (7.82)
Boys (*n* = 45)	67.84 (14.86)	25.24 (6.15)	9.56 (2.72)	44.30 (10.76)
Grade 3 (*n* − 95)				
Girls (*n* = 46)	72.10 (14.43)	25.07 (6.07)	10.86 (2.65)	47.88 (9.35)
Boys (*n* = 49)	68.49 (16.96)	25.26 (6.53)	9.27 (2.67)	45.61 (11.89)
Grade 4 (*n* = 79)				
Girls (*n* = 38)	67.79 (18.69)	24.08 (7.56)	10.36 (2.91)	44.26 (11.96)
Boys (*n* = 41)	69.77 (15.83)	25.35 (6.50)	9.83 (2.77)	45.71 (10.22)
Grade 5 (*n* = 79)				
Girls (*n* = 44)	73.02 (14.10)	26.11 (6.01)	10.76 (2.34)	48.36 (9.05)
Boys (*n* = 35)	63.68 (18.04)	23.14 (7.31)	8.69 (2.82)	42.40 (12.47)
Grade 6 (*n* = 70)				
Girls (*n* = 31)	74.10 (14.45)	26.59 (6.26)	10.79 (2.25)	48.77 (9.13)
Boys (*n* = 39)	65.24 (12.39)	23.75 (5.90)	9.05 (2.35)	43.59 (8.19)

Note. Standard deviations are in parentheses. From DuPaul, Rapport, Perriello (1991, p. 291). Copyright 1991 by the National Association of School Psychologists. Reprinted by permission.

◆◆◆

Student Interview

◆

It is important in the process of academic assessment to determine how the student being assessed perceives the demands of the academic environment. This information is best obtained through an interview of the student. Specifically, questions should cover the following: the degree to which the student understands directions of assignments; the degree of success predicted by the student on each assignment; the student's perception of how much time he/she is given by the teacher to complete assignments; the student's knowledge of how to seek assistance when experiencing difficulty; and the student's understanding of the consequences of not completing academic work. This information can be obtained by means of a semistructured interview, conducted immediately after an observation of the student engaged in an assigned task. A simple format with general guidelines is provided for conducting the interview.

Form 5

STUDENT INTERVIEW FORM

Student name _____

Subject   _____

Date   _____

STUDENT-REPORTED BEHAVIOR

_____ None completed for this area

Understands expectations of teacher	☐ Yes	☐ No	☐ Not sure
Understands assignments	☐ Yes	☐ No	☐ Not sure
Feels he/she can do the assignments	☐ Yes	☐ No	☐ Not sure
Likes the subject	☐ Yes	☐ No	☐ Not sure
Feels he/she is given enough time to complete assignments	☐ Yes	☐ No	☐ Not sure
Feels like he/she is called upon to participate in discussions	☐ Yes	☐ No	☐ Not sure

General comments:

Questions used to guide interview:

Do you think you are pretty good in _____?

If you had to pick one thing about _____ you liked, what would it be?

If you had to pick one thing about _____ you don't like, what would it be?

What do you do when you are unable to solve a problem or answer a question with your assignment in _____?

Do you enjoy working with other students when you are having trouble with your assignment in _____?

Does the teacher call on you too often? Not often enough? In _____?

♦♦♦
Direct Observation: Manual for the Behavioral Observation of Students in Schools (BOSS)

♦

Systematically observing students in classrooms is an essential part of the assessment of the instructional environment. This is true whether the referral problem is not completing assignments, having difficulties in reading, or being unable to quickly and accurately compute addition facts.

Although learning to conduct systematic observations is not difficult, it does take some concentrated practice and effort to master the method. It is a rare person (if such a person exists) who can put on a pair of skis for the first time and go schussing down the slopes of Killington. It is a rare person who can pick up a basketball and make four consecutive 3-pointers. It is a rare person who can sit down at a piano for the first time and play popular songs. It is a rare person who can get in front of a group of third-grade children and teach subtraction with regrouping. Attaining the skills to be a good skier, a good athlete, a good pianist, or a good teacher takes practice. Learning these skills calls for studying persons who are considered experts at the skills in question, trying out the new skills under supervision of such experts, receiving feedback regarding one's performance, and then practicing the newly learned skills.

This manual describes the rationale and process of direct observation. In particular, the use of the BOSS, a measure designed specifically for direct observation of academic skills, is presented.

Many thanks to Mark Fugate, PhD, for suggestions and contributions to the development of the first edition of this section of the workbook.

RATIONALE

Systematic direct observation is defined as a form of quantitative data collection. Its main purpose is numerical recording of the behaviors occurring in the observational setting. For example, if Roberta is reported as not paying attention, systematic observation may show that she was off-task 50% of the time. If Jason is reported as not completing his work, than systematic observation may find that, on average, Jason completes only two of five in-class math assignments per day. If Miguel is reported as fighting on the playground at recess, systematic observation may reveal that he was sent to the principal for fighting five times in the past 2 weeks. In each case, the use of systematic observation is an attempt to capture quantitatively the behavior actually taking place.

Of course, teachers and other professionals are constantly observing children in schools; this form of observation provides a subjective impression of a child's behavior. These impressions are important and meaningful, and can be viewed as helpful data in making sense of a child's classroom behavior. Unfortunately, although these subjective impressions are frequently accurate, they can also be inaccurate. For example, Marcus may be reported by a teacher to be a disruptive and "nasty" child due to his frequent teasing of peers. Such a report suggests that the behavior occurs frequently and should be easily observable. If asked to complete a rating scale that includes items about teasing, the teacher may report that the behavior occurs often, when, in reality, the behavior may occur rarely. However, the fact that the behavior is viewed as negative and obnoxious by the teacher may make it seem much worse than it really is. Another teacher may report that Jamie is off-task "all the time." Certainly, although Jamie's off-task behavior may be frequent, it is unlikely that she is off-task all the time. Using a form of systematic observation makes it possible to describe the teasing or levels of off-task objectively in terms of its frequency. Of course, even a low frequency of misbehavior can be very troubling; teasing that occurs once per week may be viewed as out of line and needing to be stopped. However, knowing that the problem is not as severe as one first thought may be very important in deciding how to best perceive the problem. Systematic observation of Jamie may reveal that she is actually off-task at the same rate as her peers. If that is the case, why does the teacher perceive her to have such a high frequency of inattentiveness? Using systematic observation, one can report in a more definitive way the nature of the off-task behavior that has led the teacher to develop such a perception.

There are four important reasons for conducting systematic observations. First, as already noted, getting subjective opinions about behavior is important, because these perceptions represent how important persons who deal with the problem see it; indeed, they form the basis of what we think is going on. However, subjective perceptions need to be systematically confirmed or disconfirmed. In addition, as suggested earlier, the problem may be either less or more severe than originally indicated. Thus, two important reasons for conducting systematic observation are the need to confirm or disconfirm subjective reports and to determine the exact severity of the reported problem.

A third important reason for conducting systematic observation is to provide a baseline or benchmark against which to assess the success or failure of an instructional intervention. Whenever changes in behavior occur, it is important to document the relative impact of the intervention by comparing the student's present performance with his/her performance prior to the intervention. This allows the teacher, the student, and the parents to see the gains (or losses) in performance that have occurred over time. It is also required in some states that such baseline data be obtained as part of the evaluation process.

A final reason to collect systematic observation data is to provide feedback to parties (parents, students, teachers, and other school professionals) regarding the types and levels of problems student are currently having. By using systematic observation, interested persons can actually see how behavior is changing in the classroom.

IDENTIFYING THE BEHAVIORS FOR OBSERVATION

Systematic observation requires that the behaviors to be observed be carefully and precisely defined. Behaviors that are defined too broadly may be difficult to observe accurately. At the same time, behaviors defined too narrowly may not be meaningful units of responding. The key to effectively identifying behaviors for observation is to think about which ones are likely to be the most relevant to the problem(s) of interest in the classroom.

The literature has suggested that when the problem is in the area of academics the observation of student academic engaged time is a critical variable. Strong and significant relationships have been identified between high levels of academic engagement and successful academic performance. This suggests a need for a careful analysis of the types of engagement and nonengagement that a student exhibits in classrooms (see Chapter 2 of *Academic Skills Problems, Third Edition* for a more detailed discussion).

The BOSS includes two categories of engagement and three categories of nonengagement. An additional category that examines the types of instruction occurring in the classroom is also included in the code. When the interaction of the student's engaged and nonengaged time is examined, a clear picture of the student's behavior in a context of meaningful academic outcomes can be obtained.

USE OF TECHNOLOGY IN CONDUCTING SYSTEMATIC OBSERVATION

Over the past decade, computer technology has advanced significantly to make the process of conducting systematic observations easier and much more convenient. In particular, the use of personal digital assistants (PDAs) have become increasingly popular. These handheld devices offer substantial advantages in the collection of systematic observational data. Included in the PDA is a timing device, a cueing device, a data storage system, and a data analysis system. The PDA offers an opportunity to be somewhat unobtrusive in the observation process, an important consideration when observing students during academic endeavors. In addition, because of the use of HotSync® capability, information collected on a PDA can be automatically transferred to a personal computer.

Several software programs have been developed to facilitate the collection of systematic observation on a PDA. Each of the programs offers somewhat different features, and potential users are cautioned to examine the products to find out which ones best meet their needs. The three most common products are the !Observe (*www.sopriswest.com*), the Behavioral Assessment System for Children Portable Observation System (BASC POP; *www.agsnet.org*), and the BOSS (*www.harcourtassessment.com*). The programs have different features and degrees of flexibility. In particular, the POP is tied somewhat to the observational system built into the BASC, but it does enable users to customize the observation to their own behavioral codes. The !Observe system is a fully customized system as well, not linked to any particular observation code. In contrast, the BOSS software is based primarily on collecting data in academic settings and derives the specific codes for observation from research that specifies the importance of types and nature of engaged and nonengaged academic behavior of students. The code does contain some capacity for user-defined codes, although the number of codes is somewhat limited. More important, the BOSS code, unlike other software, allows prompting of the observer through multiple modalities, has a built in feature for collecting data on a peer comparison student, and uses a system of data collection that mixes momentary and partial interval data collection that has strong research support.

A detailed description of the paper-and-pencil version of the BOSS is provided in this manual. All features of the paper-and-pencil version are also included within the software. In addition, the software provides room for user-defined codes that are not part of the paper-and-pencil version. Features of the BOSS software are also presented.

GUIDELINES FOR PAPER-AND-PENCIL DIRECT OBSERVATION

Materials

- Two sharp pencils or fine-point pens
- Clipboard
- Timing device: An interval audiotape with a tape player and earpiece (or headphones). A stopwatch is not recommended, since it can be difficult to attend both to the watch and to events in the classroom. In addition, keeping track of the interval in which the observation is taking place is critical. Use of an audiocueing device allows the observer to maintain vigilance to the classroom while simultaneously recording with accuracy.
- BOSS coding sheet(s) permitting up to 30 minutes of observation. Each minute is divided into four intervals of 15 seconds each. An observation sheet is provided for use with the BOSS, consisting of 180 intervals (60 per page) for a total of 45 minutes.

Classroom Manners

- Before observing in a classroom, the observer will need to become familiar with the daily schedule, routine, and physical layout of the classroom.
- The observer should meet briefly with the teacher before the observation to learn about classroom rules or procedures that may be in effect during the observation.
- The observer should ask the teacher the best place to sit or stand, so as to be able to observe the target student directly.
- The observer needs to have a clear view of the student, but should not be too obtrusive and should be sure to stay out of major traffic areas for other students.
- During the observation, the teacher should teach as he/she normally does.
- The observer should minimize any interactions with students or the teacher during the observation period.
- The teacher should not introduce the observer to the class when he/she arrives, but should be instructed to tell the students (prior to the observer's arrival) that someone will be coming to observe what goes on in the classroom.
- If the assessment includes working individually with the target student, it is recommended that the direct observation be conducted before the observer meets individually with the student.
- The observer's entrance into the classroom should be as naturalistic as possible. It can help if he/she enters the classroom during a natural break in the instructional routine.

MAKING A CODING INTERVAL AUDIOTAPE

Making an audiotape to use for cueing during observations is not difficult, but it does take a little time. A cueing tape for the BOSS should be at least 30 minutes in length and contain intervals of 15 seconds.

Generate a tape recording by naming aloud the intervals. Using a stopwatch and a tape recorder, the observer simply states the necessary intervals. Each interval is cued by saying, "Observe 1," "Observe 2," "Observe 3," and so forth, as each interval passes. Using the word *observe* before each number is said provides a cue that signals when the interval is about to begin. A brief statement should also be provided prior to beginning the first observation interval, such as "Get ready to observe." As the last interval on the tape ends, the observer should record an ending statement, such as "End of observation," or some other appropriate closing comment.

An advantage of saying aloud the intervals is that it provides a cue immediately before each momentary time sample observation must be made. Preparing the tape can be tedious, and if concentration is not maintained, accuracy of the tape may be compromised (i.e., each interval may not be 15 seconds in length).

Another option in developing the audiotape is simply to cue each observation interval with a specific sound (i.e., a "beep"). If the observer uses this method, it may be valuable once each minute to state the interval number, in case the observer loses track of the interval.

An advantage of the BOSS software is that the timing device is built into the PDA. Once the user specifies the interval length to be used, the PDA device will beep at each designated interval. In addition, a counter is provided that displays both the interval number and the elapsed seconds since the observations began. The loudness of the sound can be easily controlled, and for those PDAs equipped with a "vibrate" option, it is possible for the cueing device to be silent. This is an important feature if the observer is concerned about any potential distraction to students during observation. Likewise, the use of a PDA device removes the necessity of a tape recorder, earphone, clipboard, and other more obtrusive materials that are necessary to conduct the observation.

COMPLETING IDENTIFYING INFORMATION

The coding sheet used with the BOSS is included at the end of this section of the workbook. At the top of the BOSS coding sheet, the observer should be sure to write in the child's name, date, his/her own name, and the subject matter being observed. In addition, the observer is asked to note the type of instructional setting observed. The time of the observation, along with the length of the observation intervals, should also be recorded. If using the BOSS software, the user is able to set the interval length from 3 to 60 seconds, as well as the nature of the cue (low beep, high beep, vibration, or flash). The type of setting is also indicated on the BOSS software.

- *ISW:TPsnt (student in independent seatwork, teacher present)*. In this setting, the student is doing independent seatwork while the teacher is available to assist individual children. Typically, the teacher is circulating around the room.
- *ISW:TSmGP (student in independent seatwork, teacher in small group not including target student)*. This setting is marked when the target student is engaged in independent seatwork and the teacher is working with a small group that *does not* include the target student.
- *SmGp:Tled (student in small group led by teacher)*. This setting is marked when the target student is in a small group (defined as eight or fewer students) that is led by the teacher.
- *LgGp:Tled (student in large group led by teacher)*. This setting is marked when the target student is in a large group (defined as more than eight students) that is led by the teacher.
- *Other*. When "Other" is used, the type of instructional setting should be noted in the margin.

The classroom setting is marked by circling the appropriate designation. If the instructional activity changes during the course of the observation, this change should be noted on the observation form by circling the interval where the change occurred and writing in the type of setting that is now in place. All of these same data are also recorded in the opening screens of the BOSS software (see Figure 3).

FIGURE 3. Screen from the BOSS software showing session information.

OBSERVING PEER COMPARISON STUDENTS

A behavioral observation is more meaningful if the target student's behavior is compared to the same behaviors displayed by peers. The BOSS requires that data be collected not only on the target student but also on peers in the same classroom. As noted on the BOSS observation form, every fifth interval is shaded. During each of these intervals, observations are conducted on a randomly selected peer rather than the target student. Before beginning the observation, the observer should decide the sequence of peer comparison observations. For example, the observer may decide to start in the front left of the classroom and observe a different peer each fifth interval, moving down the row and then from back to front. In truth, it does not matter in which order the peer comparison data are collected. It does help, however, for the observer to have an observation plan thought out before beginning the observation of the target student.

Data from intervals in which different peers were observed are combined to derive a peer comparison score for each of the behaviors.

In the BOSS software, the peer comparison data collection process is facilitated by both an audio and visual cue that indicates to the observer that the peer should be observed. Every fifth interval, a slightly different sound occurs, and the screen flashes to a slightly different version, which is marked as the peer observation data. These cues occur automatically, and the data for the peer comparison student are calculated independently from those of the targeted student.

CODING ACADEMIC ENGAGEMENT

The BOSS divides academic engagement into two subcategories: active or passive engaged time. In either case, the student is considered to be on-task. Each of these behaviors is recorded as a momentary time sample. At the beginning of each cued interval, the observer looks at the targeted student; determines whether the student is on-task; and, if so, whether the on-task behavior constitutes an active or passive form of engagement as defined below. The occurrence of the behavior at that moment is recorded by making a mark in the appropriate box on the scoring sheet. If using the BOSS software, the observer simply touches the appropriate button (see Figure 4).

Active Engaged Time

Active engaged time (AET) is defined as those times when the student is actively attending to the assigned work. Examples of AET include the following:

- Writing
- Reading aloud
- Raising a hand
- Talking to the teacher about the assigned material
- Talking to a peer about the assigned material
- Looking up a word in a dictionary

FIGURE 4. Screen from the BOSS software showing the observation screen.

AET *should not* be scored if the student is

- Talking about nonacademic material (Verbal Off-Task)
- Walking to the worksheet bin (Motor Off-Task)
- Calling out (Verbal Off-Task), unless it is considered an appropriate response style for that classroom
- Aimlessly flipping the pages of a book (Motor Off-Task)
- Any other form of off-task behavior

Passive Engaged Time

Passive engaged time (PET) is defined as those times when the student is passively attending to assigned work. Examples of PET include the following:

- Listening to a lecture
- Looking at an academic worksheet
- Reading assigned material silently
- Looking at the blackboard during teacher instruction
- Listening to a peer respond to a question

PET *should not* be scored if the student is

- Aimlessly looking around the classroom (Passive Off-Task)
- Silently reading unassigned material (Passive Off-Task)
- Any other form of off-task behavior

At times it may be difficult to determine immediately whether the child is passively engaged or daydreaming at the first moment of an interval. In this case, it is appropriate to code passive engaged time if it becomes apparent later during that interval that the student was indeed passively engaged.

CODING NONENGAGEMENT

When a student is not engaged in academic behavior, three possible categories of off-task behavior are coded. These behaviors are recorded using a partial interval observation method. If any of the three behaviors occurs at any point during the interval, a mark is made in the appropriate box. Multiple occurrences of the same behavior within a single interval are noted only one time. If using the BOSS software, the appropriate buttons on the screen are touched.

Off-Task Motor

Off-Task Motor behaviors (OFT-M) are defined as any instance of motor activity that is not directly associated with an assigned academic task. Examples of OFT-M include the following:

- Engaging in any out-of-seat behavior (defined as buttocks not in contact with the seat)
- Aimlessly flipping the pages of a book
- Manipulating objects not related to the academic task (e.g., playing with a paper clip, throwing paper, twirling a pencil, folding paper)
- Physically touching another student when not related to an academic task
- Bending or reaching, such as picking up a pencil off the floor
- Drawing or writing that is not related to an assigned academic activity
- Turning around in one's seat, oriented away from the classroom instruction
- Fidgeting in one's seat (i.e., engaging in repetitive motor movements for at least 3 consecutive seconds; student must be off-task for this category to be scored)

OFT-M *should not* be scored if the student is

- Passing paper to a student, as instructed by the teacher
- Coloring on an assigned worksheet as instructed (AET)
- Laughing at a joke told by another student (Off-Task Verbal)
- Swinging feet while working on assigned material (AET or PET)

Off-Task Verbal

Off-Task Verbal behaviors (OFT-V) are defined as any audible verbalizations that are not permitted and/or are not related to an assigned academic task. Examples of OFT-V include the following:

- Making any audible sound, such as whistling, humming, forced burping
- Talking to another student about issues unrelated to an assigned academic task
- Talking to another student about an assigned academic task when such talk is prohibited by the teacher
- Making unauthorized comments or remarks
- Calling out answers to academic problems when the teacher has not specifically asked for an answer or permitted such behavior

OFT-V *should not* be scored if the student is

- Laughing at a joke told by the teacher
- Talking to another student about the assigned academic work during a cooperative learning group (AET)
- Calling out the answer to a problem when the teacher has permitted such behavior during instruction (AET)

Off-Task Passive

Off-Task Passive behaviors (OFT-P) are defined as those times when a student is passively not attending to an assigned academic activity for a period of at least 3 consecutive seconds. Included are those times when a student is quietly waiting after the completion of an assigned task but is not engaged in an activity authorized by the teacher. Examples of OFT-P behavior include the following:

- Sitting quietly in an unassigned activity
- Looking around the room
- Starring out the window
- Passively listening to other students talk about issues unrelated to the assigned academic activity

It is important to note that the student must be passively off-task for 3-consecutive seconds *within an interval* to be scored. Should the interval end before the full 3-second period occurs, OFT-P is not scored for that interval, and a new consecutive 3-second period is required for the next interval. For instance, suppose a student begins to stare out the window during the third interval of observation. The observer counts only 2 seconds before the fourth interval begins. The student continues to stare out the window for over 3 seconds in this interval. In this case, only the fourth interval would be scored for OFT-P. If the student had stopped staring out the window after 2 seconds of the fourth interval, then OFT-P *should not* have been scored for either interval. In addition, OFT-P *should not* be scored if the student is

- Quietly reading an assigned book (PET)
- Passively listening to other students talk about the assigned work in a cooperative learning group (PET)

CODING TEACHER-DIRECTED INSTRUCTION

Teacher-directed instruction (TDI) is coded every fifth interval, again by means of a partial interval observation method. The purpose of these observations is to provide a sampling of time in which the teacher is actively engaged in direct instruction of the classroom. TDI is defined as those times when the teacher is directly instructing the class or individuals within the class. Examples of TDI include times when the teacher is

- Instructing the whole class or group
- Demonstrating academic material at the board
- Individually assisting a student with an assigned task

TDI should not be scored if the teacher is

- Scolding the class or an individual student for misbehavior
- Giving instructions for an academic activity
- Sitting at his/her desk grading papers
- Speaking to an individual student or the class about nonacademic issues

REVIEW: PROCEDURE FOR CONDUCTING THE OBSERVATION

After the observer is seated in the classroom, he/she begins the observation by starting the audiotape or touching the start button on the screen, if using the BOSS software. The observer is cued with the words "Observe one" if using the tape, or an audible beep or vibration if using the PDA. Using the number word to indicate the beginning of each interval or the cue from the PDA, the observer immediately records at the moment that the word *one* is heard or the cue occurs, whether the student is actively or passively engaged in academic behavior. If the student is off-task at the moment that the word *one* was heard or the cue occurred, the observer leaves the boxes blank or does not touch either the AET or PET buttons. For the remainder of the interval, the observer watches to see if the student engages in any form of off-task behavior. Before the next interval begins, if the student gets out of his/her seat and then talks to another student about nonacademic issues, marks would be made in the OFT-M and OFT-V columns of interval one, or these buttons on the screen would be pushed. The BOSS software darkens the color of the button once pushed, until the interval ends. If the observer makes an error within the interval, he/she simply pushes the button again and the recording is erased. Any buttons darkened at the end of an interval are recorded in the database. The process is repeated until the observer reaches interval 5. Having decided to start with the students in the first row of desks for purposes of peer comparison data collection, upon hearing the words "Observe 5" or the peer comparison cue, the observer now looks to see whether the student sitting in the first row, left side of the room, is on-task. That student is now observed for any off-task behavior throughout the remainder of the interval. In addition, during the fifth interval, the observer records whether the teacher engaged in any directed instruction. When the sixth interval begins, the observer returns to watching and recording the behavior of the target student. This process is repeated until the observation is completed. Figure 5 displays a completed sample observation using the BOSS, and Figure 6 shows a report output for the same observation from the BOSS software.

SCORING THE BOSS

All categories of the BOSS are scored using the same metric: percentage of intervals in which the behavior occurred. Hand scoring requires that the number of intervals in which the behavior was marked as occurring be divided by the total number of intervals of observing the student, and multiplying the result by 100.

• **Step 1:** Add the number of times each behavior occurred for the target student *only*, across the rows. Enter this number on the data collection sheet in the corresponding cell under the column marked "S" (for target student). Be sure *not* to add the number of occurrences in the intervals in which peer comparison data were collected (see Figure 7).

As can be seen in Figure 7, the target student was observed to have engaged in AET for 5 out of the first 15 intervals observed, PET for 5, OFT-M for 2, OFT-V for 3, and OFT-P for 3.

• **Step 2:** Add up the number of intervals each behavior is observed for the target student across the entire observation, and record the total in the lower left portion of the form. This is done by simply adding the "S" row totals for each behavior.

BEHAVIORAL OBSERVATION OF STUDENTS IN SCHOOLS (BOSS)

Child Observed: Justin   Academic Subject: Math

Date: 9/15/03   Setting: __ ISW:TPsnt   X_ SmGp:TPsnt

Observer: JGL   __ ISW:TSmGp __ LgGp:TPsnt

Time of Observation: 10:30   Interval Length: 15   Other: _____

Moment	1	2	3	4	5*	6	7	8	9	10*	11	12	13	14	15*	S	P	T
AET	\		\		\	\	\			\		\				5	2	
PET		\						\	\		\			\	\	5	1	
Partial																		
OFT-M	\								\						\	2	1	
OFT-V						\	\			\						3	1	
OFT-P	\			\	\								\			3	1	
TDI															\			1

Moment	16	17	18	19	20*	21	22	23	24	25*	26	27	28	29	30*	S	P	T
AET	\		\								\				\	3	1	
PET			\		\	\					\					3	1	
Partial																		
OFT-M		\														1	0	
OFT-V		\								\						1	1	
OFT-P								\	\	\				\	\	5	0	
TDI					\					\					\			3

Moment	31	32	33	34	35*	36	37	38	39	40*	41	42	43	44	45*	S	P	T
AET		\			\											1	1	
PET	\		\	\							\	\	\	\		7	0	
Partial																		
OFT-M							\	\							\	2	1	
OFT-V						\	\									2	0	
OFT-P										\						0	1	
TDI										\					\			2

Moment	46	47	48	49	50*	51	52	53	54	55*	56	57	58	59	60*	S	P	T
AET					\											0	1	
PET		\	\	\						\					\	3	2	
Partial																		
OFT-M										\						1	0	
OFT-V										\	\					2	0	
OFT-P						\	\	\	\					\		5	0	
TDI															\			1

	Target Student				***Peer Comparison**			**Teacher**	
	S AET	9	% AET	18.8	S AET	5	% AET	41.7	S TDI	7
Total	S PET	18	% PET	37.5	S PET	4	% PET	33.3	% TDI	58.3
Intervals	S OFT-M	6	% OFT-M	12.5	S OFT-M	2	% OFT-M	16.7	Total Intervals
Observed	S OFT-V	8	% OFT-V	16.7	S OFT-V	2	% OFT-V	16.7	Observed 12
48	OFT-P	13	% OFT-P	27.1	S OFT-P	2	% OFT-P	16.7	

FIGURE 5. Completed BOSS observation on Justin.

BOSS RESULTS

Student: Justin P

Observer: JGL   Grade: 3

Date: 09/15/2003   Time: 9:51:27 AM   Task: Math

Setting: SmGp:TpSnt   Duration: 15 minutes   Interval:15 seconds

Behavior	Target Student		Peer Student		Teacher	
	Count	Percent	Count	Percent	Count	Percent
AET	9	18.8%	5	41.7%	–	–
PET	18	37.5%	4	33.3%	–	–
OFT-M	6	12.5%	2	16.7%	–	–
OFT-V	8	16.7%	2	16.7%	–	–
OFT-P	13	27.1%	2	16.7%	–	–
TDI	–	–	–	–	7	58.3%
	Target Ints 48				Peer/Teacher Ints 12	

	AET	PET	OFT-M	OFT-V	OFT-P	TDI
1	1	0	1	0	1	–
2	0	1	0	0	0	–
3	1	0	0	0	0	–
4	0	0	0	0	1	–
5	1	0	0	0	1	0
6	1	0	0	1	0	–
7	1	0	0	1	0	–
8	0	1	0	0	0	–
9	0	1	1	0	0	–
10	1	0	0	1	0	0
11	0	1	0	1	0	–
12	1	0	0	0	0	–
13	0	0	0	0	1	–
14	0	1	0	0	0	–
15	0	1	1	0	0	1
16	1	0	0	0	0	–
17	0	0	1	1	0	–
18	0	1	0	0	0	–
19	1	0	0	0	0	–
20	0	1	0	0	0	1
21	0	1	0	0	0	–
22	0	0	0	0	1	–
23	0	0	0	0	1	–
24	0	0	0	0	1	–
25	0	0	0	1	0	1
26	1	0	0	0	0	–
27	0	1	0	0	0	–
28	0	0	0	0	1	–
29	0	0	0	0	1	–
30	1	0	0	0	0	1
31	0	1	0	0	0	–
32	1	0	0	0	0	–
33	0	1	0	0	0	–
34	0	1	0	0	0	–
35	1	0	0	0	0	0
36	0	0	0	1	0	–

FIGURE 6. Report generated from the BOSS software for Justin P.

	AET	PET	OFT-M	OFT-V	OFT-P	TDI
37	0	0	0	1	0	–
38	0	0	1	0	0	–
39	0	0	1	0	0	–
40	*0*	*0*	*0*	*0*	*1*	*1*
41	0	1	0	0	0	–
42	0	1	0	0	0	–
43	0	1	0	0	0	–
44	0	1	0	0	0	–
45	*0*	*0*	*1*	*0*	*0*	*1*
46	0	0	0	0	0	–
47	0	1	0	0	0	–
48	0	1	0	0	0	–
49	0	1	0	0	0	–
50	*1*	*0*	*0*	*0*	*0*	*0*
51	0	0	0	0	1	–
52	0	0	0	0	1	–
53	0	0	0	0	1	–
54	0	0	0	0	1	–
55	*0*	*1*	*0*	*0*	*0*	*0*
56	0	0	1	1	0	–
57	0	0	0	1	0	–
58	0	0	0	0	0	–
59	0	0	0	0	1	–
60	*0*	*1*	*0*	*0*	*0*	*1*

Behavior Legend

AET	Actively Engaged in Task
PET	Passively Engaged in Task
OFT-M	Off-Task Motor
OFT-V	Off-Task Verbal
OFT-P	Off-Task Passive
TDI	Teacher-Directed Instruction

FIGURE 6. *(continued)*

As can be seen in Figure 5, the target student was found to engage in AET for 9 intervals, PET for 18 intervals, OFT-M for 6 intervals, OFT-V for 8 intervals, and OFT-P for 13 intervals.

• **Step 3:** Determine the total number of intervals in which the target student was observed, and record this number in the space provided in the lower left portion of the data collection sheet. Again, be sure to eliminate any intervals in which the peer comparison data were collected.

As evident in Figure 5, the target student was observed for a total of 48 intervals during this observation.

• **Step 4:** Divide the number of occurrences of each behavior by the total intervals observed and multiply by 100. This is the percentage of intervals in which the behavior was observed to occur. Record this in the spaces provided.

• **Step 5:** Repeat this process, but now calculate only the intervals in which

Moment	1	2	3	4	5*	6	7	8	9	10*	11	12	13	14	15*	S	P	T
AET	\		\		\	\	\			\		\				5		
PET		\						\	\		\			\	\	5		
Partial																		
OFT-M	\								\						\	2		
OFT-V						\	\			\	\					3		
OFT-P	\			\	\								\			3		
TDI					\									\				

FIGURE 7. First 15 intervals of BOSS observation for Justin.

peer comparison data (P) were collected. Eliminate any intervals in which the target student was observed (see Figure 8).

• **Step 6:** Repeat the process one more time, but now examine only the intervals in which TDI data were collected (see Figure 9). Eliminate any intervals in which the target the student data were collected. Note that the intervals in which peer comparison data were collected are the same ones in which TDI is observed.

In the example shown in Figure 5, the target student was observed for a total of 48 intervals, peers for 12 intervals. Across the observation, AET for the target student was observed nine times, resulting in 18.8% of the intervals. For the peer comparison students, AET was observed five times out of 12 intervals, or 41.7% of the intervals. Calculations for all categories should result in the summary on the bottom of Figure 5.

If an observer is using the BOSS software, all of these calculations are automatically provided at the end of the observation and displayed on the PDA. The data are automatically stored and transferred to a personal computer through the HotSync process. A report is then generated based on the observation (see Figure 6).

INTERPRETATION OF BOSS DATA

Interpretation of the BOSS data can involve analysis of several aspects of classroom behavior. First, the BOSS shows the levels of academic engagement and non-

Moment	1	2	3	4	5*	6	7	8	9	10*	11	12	13	14	15*	S	P	T
AET	\		\		\	\	\			\		\				5	2	
PET		\						\	\		\			\	\	5	1	
Partial																		
OFT-M	\								\						\	2	1	
OFT-V						\	\			\	\					3	1	
OFT-P	\			\	\								\			3	1	
TDI					\									\				

FIGURE 8. First 15 intervals of BOSS observation for Justin scored for peer comparison students.

Moment	1	2	3	4	5*	6	7	8	9	10*	11	12	13	14	15*	S	P	T
AET	\		\		\	\	\			\		\				5	2	
PET		\						\	\		\			\	\	5	1	
Partial																		
OFT-M	\							\							\	2	1	
OFT-V						\	\			\	\					3	1	
OFT-P	\			\	\								\			3	1	
TDI					\										\			2

FIGURE 9. First 15 intervals of BOSS observation for Justin scored for TDI.

engagement for the targeted student in the particular setting of observation. By comparing the combined percentages of AET and PET against those of the three OFT categories, the observer can establish the amount of a student's on- and off-task behavior. These data can provide the observer with information about the extent to which the target student is effectively engaged in the learning process.

Second, observations across multiple settings make it possible to determine relative differences in the target student's academic engagement in different instructional environments. For example, it may be found that a student has much higher levels of on-task behavior when he/she is in a teacher-led setting than when involved in independent seatwork.

Third, by examining the relative differences between AET and PET, the observer can determine whether the opportunities to respond (AET level) for a student are high enough to provide clear evidence of academic progress. Students who are struggling in school are often found to have relatively low levels of AET even when they are on-task.

Fourth, and most importantly, the observer can compare the performance of the target student against the student's peers. Use of this type of local normative data is crucial in understanding the degree to which the levels of behavior obtained for the target student differ from the expected performance of the student's classmates. At times, a student who appears to have very low levels of on-task behavior may be found to have a level equivalent to those of his/her peers, suggesting that the student's behavior may not be beyond the expectations set by the classroom teacher. On the other hand, a student appearing to have very high levels of on-task behavioral performance may be viewed as not meeting classroom expectations. When comparisons are made to the student's peers, it may become evident that although the student's level is high, it is significantly lower than the levels of his/her peers.

One of the most frequently asked questions related to conducting systematic observation is, "How much observation is needed?" The answer is, "It depends." Accurate observations require at least 10–15 minutes. Optimally, observations should be 20–30 minutes each. In the best of all possible worlds, the observation should be repeated over 2–3 days, and possibly across different types of academic settings (e.g., independent work in reading, small-group activities in math, large-group activities in science, etc.). Obviously, the practical restrictions of time may limit how much observation can be done. So the question is whether a single observation can be enough.

The key to good observation is that it accurately represents the child's behavior at the time of the observation and at other times of the day. If a child's behavior tends to be highly variable from day to day or hour to hour, a single observation at one time in one setting may not be sufficient. Likewise, if a child's behavior changes because there is an observer in the classroom, or the child is having a "good day," a single observation may not be enough. Certainly, some degree of stable responding from day to day is important; however, the problem of some children is precisely that they are inconsistent, so expecting consistency in those cases is unrealistic.

One way to address this problem is always to ask the teacher whether the behavior seen that day was typical of the student's performance. If it was, then the one observation may be enough. However, if the child's behavior was atypical of what the teacher thinks is his/her usual behavior, than additional observations are needed.

Another important issue to consider in deciding whether enough observation has been done is whether the situation in which the behavior was observed represents where the problems tend to occur. For example, although the teacher notes that Josh has problems during independent seatwork activities, an important question for the teacher is whether there are equal problems in math or reading. One hypothesis about Josh's behavior may be that his skill levels differ across subject matter, and the differential skill levels result in differential behavioral outcomes. Thus, it may be crucial to conduct observations during independent seatwork periods in both a math and reading activity.

The rule of thumb often recommended is that observers should plan to conduct at least three observations. If behavior is consistent after two observations, than the third can perhaps be bypassed. If the behavior is not consistent after three observations, than at least one additional observation should be conducted. It is important to note that the decision about when enough observation has been conducted must be a clinical decision made from sound clinical judgment. There is no single rule that can be applied in all cases.

In the example shown in Figure 5, the student, Justin, was observed during his math class. Throughout the observation, the teacher was engaged in teaching a small group (six students) in which Justin was included. Peer comparison data for this observation were collected among the other five students in Justin's small group. The observation lasted for 15 minutes and was conducted at 10:30 A.M. Justin's overall level of on-task behavior is much lower than that of his peers. In total, Justin was academically engaged for 56.3% of the observed intervals, while his peers remained engaged for 75.0% of the observed intervals. In addition, when Justin was engaged, he spent the largest proportion of his time (37.5% of the intervals) in passive rather than active forms of engagement. In contrast, his peers were actively engaged for 41.7% of the intervals.

When Justin was off-task, he was primarily nonengaged in passive ways. Typically, this involved looking away from his work and staring out the windows. Justin was also off-task through getting out of his seat, as well as speaking to his peers. However, these off-task behaviors for Justin were comparable to those of his classmates.

Throughout the observation, Justin's teacher was engaged in directed teaching activities for approximately 58.3% of the observed intervals. During intervals when

Justin's teacher was not instructing the class, she was observed in classroom management activities, such as redirecting Justin and other students to pay attention to her direction.

In regard to interpreting data from the BOSS, it is important to note that the observer does not view the level of behavior obtained through the observation to represent an estimate of the amount of time that a behavior would occur. Because the observation system is derived from a time-sampling strategy, it would be inaccurate to say that the behavior occurred for __% of the time. This is especially true since partial interval recording systems (such as those used here for the off-task behaviors and TDI) are likely to overestimate the actual rate of a behavior's occurrence. It is also important to note that the data collected for the target student are likely to be more reliable and stable then the data collected for peer comparison purposes. The more observation intervals, the better the stability of the measure. In this observation example, there were 48 observations of the target student and only 12 of the peers. Data collected on peers must be considered cautiously in the interpretation of results.

Form 6

BEHAVIORAL OBSERVATION OF STUDENTS IN SCHOOLS (BOSS)

Child Observed: _____   Academic Subject: _____

Date: _____   Setting: __ ISW:TPsnt   __ SmGp:TPsnt

Observer: _____   __ ISW:TSmGp __ LgGp:TPsnt

Time of Observation: _____   Interval Length: _____   Other: _____

Moment	1	2	3	4	5*	6	7	8	9	10*	11	12	13	14	15*	S	P	T
AET																		
PET																		
Partial																		
OFT-M																		
OFT-V																		
OFT-P																		
TDI																		

Moment	16	17	18	19	20*	21	22	23	24	25*	26	27	28	29	30*	S	P	T
AET																		
PET																		
Partial																		
OFT-M																		
OFT-V																		
OFT-P																		
TDI																		

Moment	31	32	33	34	35*	36	37	38	39	40*	41	42	43	44	45*	S	P	T
AET																		
PET																		
Partial																		
OFT-M																		
OFT-V																		
OFT-P																		
TDI																		

Moment	46	47	48	49	50*	51	52	53	54	55*	56	57	58	59	60*	S	P	T
AET																		
PET																		
Partial																		
OFT-M																		
OFT-V																		
OFT-P																		
TDI																		

	Target Student			*Peer Comparison			Teacher	
	S AET _____	% AET _____		S AET _____	% AET _____		S TDI _____	
Total	S PET _____	% PET _____		S PET _____	% PET _____		% TDI _____	
Intervals	S OFT-M _____	% OFT-M _____		S OFT-M _____	% OFT-M _____		Total Intervals	
Observed	S OFT-V _____	% OFT-V _____		S OFT-V _____	% OFT-V _____		Observed _____	
	OFT-P _____	% OFT-P _____		S OFT-P _____	% OFT-P _____			

BEHAVIORAL OBSERVATION OF STUDENTS IN SCHOOLS (BOSS)

Child Observed: _____   Academic Subject: _____

Date: _____   Setting: ___ ISW:TPsnt   ___ SmGp:TPsnt

Observer: _____   ___ ISW:TSmGp   ___ LgGp:TPsnt

Time of Observation: _____   Interval Length: _____   Other: _____

Moment	61	62	63	64	65*	66	67	68	69	70*	71	72	73	74	75*	S	P	T
AET																		
PET																		
Partial																		
OFT-M																		
OFT-V																		
OFT-P																		
TDI																		

Moment	76	77	78	79	80*	81	82	83	84	85*	86	87	88	89	90*	S	P	T
AET																		
PET																		
Partial																		
OFT-M																		
OFT-V																		
OFT-P																		
TDI																		

Moment	91	92	93	94	95*	96	97	98	99	100*	101	102	103	104	105*	S	P	T
AET																		
PET																		
Partial																		
OFT-M																		
OFT-V																		
OFT-P																		
TDI																		

Moment	106	107	108	109	110*	111	112	113	114	115*	116	117	118	119	120*	S	P	T
AET																		
PET																		
Partial																		
OFT-M																		
OFT-V																		
OFT-P																		
TDI																		

	Target Student		*Peer Comparison		Teacher
	S AET _____ % AET _____	S AET _____ % AET _____	S TDI _____
Total	S PET _____ % PET _____	S PET _____ % PET _____	% TDI _____
Intervals	S OFT-M _____ % OFT-M _____	S OFT-M _____ % OFT-M _____	Total Intervals
Observed	S OFT-V _____ % OFT-V _____	S OFT-V _____ % OFT-V _____	Observed _____
_____	OFT-P _____ % OFT-P _____	S OFT-P _____ % OFT-P _____	

51

BEHAVIORAL OBSERVATION OF STUDENTS IN SCHOOLS (BOSS)

Child Observed: _____

Date: _____

Observer: _____

Time of Observation: _____

Academic Subject: _____

Setting: ___ ISW:TPsnt ___ SmGp:TPsnt

___ ISW:TSmGp ___ LgGp:TPsnt

Interval Length: _____ Other: _____

Moment	121	122	123	124	125*	126	127	128	129	130*	131	132	133	134	135*	S	P	T
AET																		
PET																		
Partial																		
OFT-M																		
OFT-V																		
OFT-P																		
TDI																		

Moment	136	137	138	139	140*	141	142	143	144	145*	146	147	148	149	150*	S	P	T
AET																		
PET																		
Partial																		
OFT-M																		
OFT-V																		
OFT-P																		
TDI																		

Moment	151	152	153	154	155*	156	157	158	159	160*	161	162	163	164	165*	S	P	T
AET																		
PET																		
Partial																		
OFT-M																		
OFT-V																		
OFT-P																		
TDI																		

Moment	166	167	168	169	170*	171	172	173	174	175*	176	177	178	179	180*	S	P	T
AET																		
PET																		
Partial																		
OFT-M																		
OFT-V																		
OFT-P																		
TDI																		

	Target Student		*Peer Comparison		Teacher
	S AET _____	% AET _____	S AET _____	% AET _____	S TDI _____
Total	S PET _____	% PET _____	S PET _____	% PET _____	% TDI _____
Intervals	S OFT-M _____	% OFT-M _____	S OFT-M _____	% OFT-M _____	Total Intervals
Observed	S OFT-V _____	% OFT-V _____	S OFT-V _____	% OFT-V _____	Observed _____
_____	OFT-P _____	% OFT-P _____	S OFT-P _____	% OFT-P _____	

STEP 2

♦♦♦

Assessing Instructional Placement

♦

◆◆◆
Reading
◆

In a direct assessment of reading, the oral reading rate is typically the metric used to assess student progress. However, this metric is only one of several that can be used for conducting a curriculum-based assessment of reading. When the examiner is interested in using a metric that may be more sensitive to changes in comprehension skills, two measures that may have value are the use of a cloze technique and an oral retell technique. A cloze technique presents students with a reading passage in which certain words are eliminated; the student's task is to supply the missing words. Fuchs, Hamlett, and Fuchs (1999b) have developed a computer program (available from Pro-Ed, *www.proedinc.com*) that provides a modified cloze technique, called a maze, in which the student is provided with a choice of three possible words, only one of which makes sense in the paragraph. Although only available for the Macintosh series computers, the program has been shown to be a potentially accurate method for monitoring progress in reading over time (Fuchs & Fuchs, 1992). Interested readers should consult both the Fuchs and Fuchs article and the computer program for detailed descriptions of this modified cloze technique.

A similar maze measure for assessing reading comprehension has also been developed by AIMSweb® (*www.aimsweb.com*). The AIMSweb product is a paper-and-pencil version of the technique developed by Fuchs et al. (1999b), with grade-level reading passages for grades 1–8. Beginning with the second sentence, every seventh word is removed, with three choices available for the student. One of the words is correct, another is a closely related but incorrect response, and still another is a distracter. Students are asked to circle the correct word as they read the passage. They are given 3 minutes to read the passage, and the number of correct maze words per minute represents the score on the item. Figure 10 provides an example

Jason and Max picked next Friday to carry out their special mission. Friday was a week away. They **(agreed, had, branches)** so many things to accomplish. In **(plan, order, at)** to reach their final goal, the **(next, branches, boys)** made a plan for each day **(to, of, each)** the week. They had to work **(hard, creek, big)** every day to finish each task. **(Pile, Could, Had)** they do it all?

On Monday, **(creek, big, they)** agreed to meet and put plan **(near, wood, A)** into action. Plan A was to **(gather, work, day)** as many fallen branches as they **(could, on, had)** carry. They hauled the wood from **(neat, a, the)** edge of the cornfield and stacked **(agree, it, they)** in a big pile at the **(plan, edge, hauled)** of the forest.

On Tuesday, the **(rocks, by, boys)** met near the lazy creek and **(put, climb, wood)** plan B into motion. They dug **(up, near, the)** rocks the size of footballs from **(and, night, the)** creek's bottom. By dusk, they had **(rode, arranged, to)** the rocks in a neat circle **(a, next, up)** to the pile of branches they **(their, found, had)** hauled the night before.

On Wednesday, **(plan, the, work)** C was to climb into the **(attic, umbrellas, they)** above Jason's garage. They searched around **(Max, in, with)** flashlights and both found backpacks. They **(spoke, under, wore)** their packs as they rode their **(without, bikes, garage)** to the edge of the forest **(to, end, for)** complete the day's work.

On Thursday **(they, it, work)** rained. They had to drop the **(up, plan, forest)** for the day. Still, Jason and **(went, backpack, Max)** met at the end of their **(bikes, driveways, on)** under umbrellas. They quietly spoke. They **(rained, decided, tent)** their mission would work without plan **(D, fire, was)**.

When the sun went down on **(only, Friday, evening)**, they met at the edge of **(the, out, and)** forest. There sat their tent. They'd **(stacked, tasks, set)** it up on Wednesday evening. The **(circle, special, wood)** was ready to go into their **(campfire, many, night)** ring. Their next step was to **(big, build, climb)** a warm fire:

The mission to **(camp, step, the)** out was complete. The only tasks **(Max, now, next)** were to sit back and enjoy **(a, the, ring)** fruits of their labor.

Jason and Max picked next Friday to carry out their special mission. Friday was a week away. They **(had)** so many things to accomplish. In **(order)** to reach their final goal, the **(boys)** made a plan for each day **(of)** the week. They had to work **(hard)** every day to finish each task. **(Could)** they do it all?

On Monday, **(they)** agreed to meet and put plan **(A)** into action. Plan A was to **(gather)** as many fallen branches as they **(could)** carry. They hauled the wood from **(the)** edge of the cornfield and stacked **(it)** in a big pile at the **(edge)** of the forest.

On Tuesday, the **(boys)** met near the lazy creek and **(put)** plan B into motion. They dug **(up)** rocks the size of footballs from **(the)** creek's bottom. By dusk, they had **(arranged)** the rocks in a neat circle **(next)** to the pile of branches they **(had)** hauled the night before.

On Wednesday, **(plan)** C was to climb into the **(attic)** above Jason's garage. They searched around **(with)** flashlights and both found backpacks. They **(wore)** their packs as they rode their **(bikes)** to the edge of the forest **(to)** complete the day's work.

On Thursday **(it)** rained. They had to drop the **(plan)** for the day. Still, , Jason and **(Max)** met at the end of their **(driveways)** under umbrellas. They quietly spoke. They **(decided)** their mission would work without plan **(D)**.

When the sun went down on **(Friday)**, they met at the edge of **(the)** forest. There sat their tent. They'd **(set)** it up on Wednesday evening. The **(wood)** was ready to go into their **(campfire)** ring. Their next step was to **(build)** a warm fire.

The mission to **(camp)** out was complete. The only tasks **(now)** were to sit back and enjoy **(the)** fruits of their labor.

FIGURE 10. Example of Maze task for grade 3 from AIMSweb. Copyright 2002 by Edformation, Inc. Reprinted by permission.

from the AIMSweb product of a paper-and-pencil version of the maze technique. No clear benchmarks for typical performance of students on this measure have been developed at this time. Individuals who decide to use the maze measure should probably conduct a local norm to establish benchmarks for performance across typical students.

The use of oral retell techniques may also be a valuable adjunct to a curriculum-based assessment of reading. In this technique, students are asked to read a passage and then retell the story in their own words. The task can be done using silent and oral reading if the evaluator suspects that a student is having difficulties when asked to read aloud. The student's responses can be scored using a checklist or rating scale such as that provided in Form 7. This particular form is useful for narrative passages, but a similar type of checklist can be developed for more expository text.

ORAL RETELL TECHNIQUE

- **Step 1:** The examiner selects a passage for the student to read. The passage should be between 250 and 300 words for a student in grade 3 or above, or between 150 and 200 words for a student in grades 1–2. The passage used should also have a story or theme embedded in it.
- **Step 2:** The examiner asks the student read the entire passage aloud, and times the reading (first minute only) to determine the rate of words read correctly and incorrectly per minute.
- **Step 3:** The examiner then asks the student to retell the story in his/her own words, and tape-records the response for later scoring. The retell should be done in the following sequence: If the student is able to complete the retell accurately accordingly to Level A procedures, then Levels B, C, and D would not be done. The examiner should proceed to the next level of the retell technique if the student is unsuccessful at the preceding level.

  - Level A: *Nonprompted retell without passage.* The examiner asks the student to retell, without allowing him/her access to the passage. When the student cannot add anything else to his/her retell, he/she is stopped.
  - Level B: *Nonprompted retell with passage.* The examiner asks the student to retell, allowing him/her access to the passage. Again, when the student cannot add anything to the retell, he/she is stopped.
  - Level C: *Prompted retell without passage.* The examiner does not allow the student access to the passage but provides the student with a simple prompt about the story. For example, for the story described in the case example below, the evaluator might ask the student, "The main idea of this story was about a circus coming to town. Now tell me more about the story." The examiner can continue to prompt the student to see how many prompts are needed in order for the student to accurately recall the information read. The student is stopped when he/she cannot recall anything further.
  - Level D: *Prompted retell with access to passage.* The student is allowed to

look at the passage as the examiner provides a simple prompt about the story. For example, for this story, the evaluator might say to the student, "The main idea of this story was about a circus coming to town. Now tell me more about the story." Again, the examiner can continue to prompt the student to see how many prompts are needed in order for the student to accurately recall the information read. The student is stopped when he/she cannot recall anything further.

• **Step 4:** The examiner scores the retell against the retelling scoring form provided or developed for the passage. Again, an example of such a scoring form is provided below.

Another variation of the retell technique would ask the student to read the story silently to him/herself rather than aloud.

QUANTIFICATION OF RETELLING FOR NARRATIVE TEXT

Student's Name: _____

Book/Page: _____   Date: _____

Directions: Place a 1 next to each item the student includes in his/her retelling. Credit the gist, as well as the obvious recall. Place an * if you ask the child questions to aid recall.

		Level				
		A	B	C	D	
Story sense						
Theme:	Main idea or moral of story	☐	☐	☐	☐	(1)
Problem:	Difficulty to overcome	☐	☐	☐	☐	(1)
Goal:	What the character wants to happen	☐	☐	☐	☐	(1)
Title:	Name of the story (if possible)	☐	☐	☐	☐	(1)
Setting						
	When and where the story occurs	☐	☐	☐	☐	(1)
Characters						
	Name the main characters	☐	☐	☐	☐	(1)
Events/episodes						
	Initiating event	☐	☐	☐	☐	(1)
	Major events (climax)	☐	☐	☐	☐	(1)
	Sequence: retells in structural order	☐	☐	☐	☐	(1)
Resolution						
	Name problem solution for the goal	☐	☐	☐	☐	(.5)
	End the story	☐	☐	☐	☐	(.5)

TOTAL ___ ___ ___ ___

RETELL TECHNIQUE: EXAMPLES AND EXERCISES

Case Descriptions

Shawn was a fourth-grade student in a general education classroom. He was selected by his teacher as an average-performing student in her classroom. Troy was a fourth-grade student in the same general education classroom as Shawn. His teacher selected him as a student having significant problems in reading in her class. Both students were asked to read the following passage and then to retell the story in their own words, without use of the passage (Level A retell). After reading each student's retell, readers are invited to complete the Quantification of Retelling form provided for each one. A completed form is provided on the following page in each case.

Passage Read

The people of Lone Tree, Texas, often wonder why the circus never comes to their town. Almost nobody remembers the one time, years ago, that the circus did come to town.

Lone Tree was a busy cowtown. Two trains stopped there each day. On Saturday night folks from miles around came to town—ranchers, cowboys, Indians, and homesteaders. Bearpaw Smith's store had just about everything that the people needed. But there was one thing missing. None of these people had ever seen the circus.

Then one day a silent stranger came to Lone Tree and plastered the walls of Bearpaw Smith's store with circus posters. The circus was coming to town! The people were so excited, they could hardly wait for the day of the show. The big day finally arrived, and it would be a day to remember.

An hour before showtime the crowd on the midway and around the ticket wagon was already so great that it seemed impossible that the circus tent would be able to hold them all. And still the people came.

One of the latecomers was Clyde Jones, the mountain-lion hunter, with his pack of "lion hounds." The circus people said it was against the rules to take dogs into the tent. Clyde said his were the best hounds in the state and where he went they went. The ticket taker answered that this was one place they were not going to go. If Clyde wanted to see the circus, he'd have to leave his dogs outside. Clyde grumbled but he did want to see the circus, so he tied the hounds to tent stakes and left them howling after him as he went inside.

Results of Retelling for Shawn

Rates: Words correct/minute = 131
                  Words incorrect/minute = 0

Verbatim transcript: "It's about a town in Texas, and they've never seen, like, a circus before, and they want to see it. And they know a store that has everything except for a circus. And one day the store gets plastered, and they find out there is going to be a circus coming, and when they see it they can't believe that everyone can all fit into the tent. And then there is a man that comes late and he has, like, hounds and he can't bring them in, so he just leaves them out. But he wanted to bring them in, but he had to leave them outside."

Instructions: On page 62, score Shawn's retelling for Level A before looking at the scored form on page 63.

QUANTIFICATION OF RETELLING FOR NARRATIVE TEXT

Student's Name: _____

Book/Page: _____ Date: _____

Directions: Place a 1 next to each item the student includes in his/her retelling. Credit the gist, as well as the obvious recall. Place an * if you ask the child questions to aid recall.

		Level				
		A	B	C	D	
Story sense						
Theme:	Main idea or moral of story	☐	☐	☐	☐	(1)
Problem:	Difficulty to overcome	☐	☐	☐	☐	(1)
Goal:	What the character wants to happen	☐	☐	☐	☐	(1)
Title:	Name of the story (if possible)	☐	☐	☐	☐	(1)
Setting						
	When and where the story occurs	☐	☐	☐	☐	(1)
Characters						
	Name the main characters	☐	☐	☐	☐	(1)
Events/episodes						
	Initiating event	☐	☐	☐	☐	(1)
	Major events (climax)	☐	☐	☐	☐	(1)
	Sequence: retells in structural order	☐	☐	☐	☐	(1)
Resolution						
	Name problem solution for the goal	☐	☐	☐	☐	(.5)
	End the story	☐	☐	☐	☐	(.5)

TOTAL ___ ___ ___ ___

Exercise 1: Scored Form for Shawn

QUANTIFICATION OF RETELLING FOR NARRATIVE TEXT

Student's Name: _Shawn_

Book/Page: _____   Date: _____

Directions: Place a 1 next to each item the student includes in his/her retelling. Credit the gist, as well as the obvious recall. Place an * if you ask the child questions to aid recall.

Level

			A	B	C	D	
Story sense							
Theme:	Main idea or moral of story		☒	☐	☐	☐	(1)
Problem:	Difficulty to overcome		☒	☐	☐	☐	(1)
Goal:	What the character wants to happen		☒	☐	☐	☐	(1)
Title:	Name of the story (if possible)		☐	☐	☐	☐	(1)
Setting							
	When and where the story occurs		☒	☐	☐	☐	(1)
Characters							
	Name the main characters		☐	☐	☐	☐	(1)
Events/episodes							
	Initiating event		☒	☐	☐	☐	(1)
	Major events (climax)		☒	☐	☐	☐	(1)
	Sequence: retells in structural order		☒	☐	☐	☐	(1)
Resolution							
	Name problem solution for the goal		☒	☐	☐	☐	(.5)
	End the story		☒	☐	☐	☐	(.5)

TOTAL __8__ ___ ___ ___

Comment: Note that Shawn's performance at Level A suggests no need to move to other levels of the retell technique.

Results of Retelling for Troy

Rates: Words correct/minute = 55
                 Errors/minute = 3

Verbatim transcript: (*Long pause.*) "The people are saying there has never been a circus in town before. So one day they heard there was a circus coming to town. Everybody was so happy they couldn't wait for the day to come. (*Examiner: Anything else?*) No."

Instructions: On page 65, score Troy's retelling for Level A before looking at the scored form on page 66.

QUANTIFICATION OF RETELLING FOR NARRATIVE TEXT

Student's Name: _____

Book/Page: _____ Date: _____

Directions: Place a 1 next to each item the student includes in his/her retelling. Credit the gist, as well as the obvious recall. Place an * if you ask the child questions to aid recall.

		Level	
		A B C D	

Story sense
Theme:	Main idea or moral of story	☐ ☐ ☐ ☐	(1)
Problem:	Difficulty to overcome	☐ ☐ ☐ ☐	(1)
Goal:	What the character wants to happen	☐ ☐ ☐ ☐	(1)
Title:	Name of the story (if possible)	☐ ☐ ☐ ☐	(1)

Setting
| | When and where the story occurs | ☐ ☐ ☐ ☐ | (1) |

Characters
| | Name the main characters | ☐ ☐ ☐ ☐ | (1) |

Events/episodes
	Initiating event	☐ ☐ ☐ ☐	(1)
	Major events (climax)	☐ ☐ ☐ ☐	(1)
	Sequence: retells in structural order	☐ ☐ ☐ ☐	(1)

Resolution
| | Name problem solution for the goal | ☐ ☐ ☐ ☐ | (.5) |
| | End the story | ☐ ☐ ☐ ☐ | (.5) |

TOTAL ___ ___ ___ ___

Exercise 2: Scored Form for Troy
QUANTIFICATION OF RETELLING FOR NARRATIVE TEXT

Student's Name: _Troy_____

Book/Page: _____ Date: _____

Directions: Place a 1 next to each item the student includes in his/her retelling. Credit the gist, as well as the obvious recall. Place an * if you ask the child questions to aid recall.

			Level				
			A	B	C	D	
Story sense							
	Theme:	Main idea or moral of story	☒	☐	☐	☐	(1)
	Problem:	Difficulty to overcome	☐	☐	☐	☐	(1)
	Goal:	What the character wants to happen	☐	☐	☐	☐	(1)
	Title:	Name of the story (if possible)	☐	☐	☐	☐	(1)
Setting		When and where the story occurs	☐	☐	☐	☐	(1)
Characters		Name the main characters	☐	☐	☐	☐	(1)
Events/episodes		Initiating event	☒	☐	☐	☐	(1)
		Major events (climax)	☐	☐	☐	☐	(1)
		Sequence: retells in structural order	☐	☐	☐	☐	(1)
Resolution		Name problem solution for the goal	☐	☐	☐	☐	(.5)
		End the story	☐	☐	☐	☐	(.5)

TOTAL _2_ ___ ___ ___

Comment: Given the poor performance of Troy, the examiner would continue through the levels of prompted retell.

Math

One of the key aspects of curriculum-based assessment of math is using "digits correct per minute" or "total digits" as a metric in the scoring of student performance. In addition, in order to develop more effective interventions, examiners need to be able to conduct an analysis of the types of errors students are making as they complete the math probes. This section of the workbook provides descriptions of how to score math probes using digits correct per minute, along with examples of conducting an analysis of errors. Practice exercises for both scoring and interpretation of math probes are included.

A second component to curriculum-based assessment of math is the evaluation of student performance on measures of mathematical concepts–applications. Scoring these types of measures is not complex; however, developing these types of measures can be quite time-consuming. An example of this type of measure, along with its scoring, is provided, with indications where readers can obtain commercial measures of mathematics concepts–applications.

USING DIGITS CORRECT IN SCORING MATH PROBES

Typically, when a student is asked to complete math problems, the teacher marks the student's response as either correct or incorrect. Even small and minor errors in the computation process result in the student's obtaining an incorrect answer. In assessing the outcomes of an instructional process, an examiner needs to use a metric that across time can be sensitive to the student's gradual acquisition of the skills required to complete computations accurately. The metric digits correct rather than problems correct accomplishes this goal.

For example, a student asked to add two three-digit numbers may initially get 0 digits correct:

(1)   356
                                           + 678
                                            922

Recognizing the student's lack of knowledge of regrouping principles, the teacher begins to teach the student how to regroup from the 1's to the 10's column. After some instruction, the student now does the following when given a similar type of problem:

(2)   467
                                           + 589
                                            946

This problem shows the student to have one digit correct. After additional instruction, the student produces the results of problem (3):

(3)   378
                                           + 657
                                            1035

The metric of digits correct makes evident the student's gradual acquisition of the regrouping concept. If the evaluator were to use only the problem's correctness or incorrectness to determine whether the student was learning the concept of regrouping, the student's gradual acquisition of the skill would not be evident.

SCORING DIGITS CORRECT
FOR ADDITION AND SUBTRACTION PROBLEMS

The calculation of digits correct when the student is completing addition or subtraction problems is fairly straightforward. Each correct digit <u>below</u> the answer line is counted. If the problem involves regrouping, and the student places numbers above the columns to indicate how much was carried to the next column, these numbers are not counted in the digits-correct figure.

   Examples:

          12   145
        + 4   + 672
          16 (2 digits correct)   817 (3 digits correct)

          54   2675
        − 27   − 1089
          27 (2 digits correct)   1586 (4 digits correct)

In a math curriculum-based assessment, sets of problems are administered under timed conditions, and a calculation is made of the number of digits correct per minute. Exercise 3 provides an opportunity to practice scoring addition and subtraction math problems using digits correct per minute.

Exercise 3
DIGITS CORRECT FOR ADDITION AND SUBTRACTION PROBLEMS

Addition and Subtraction Facts with Regrouping to 10's Column

A	B	C	D	E
15 − 9 —— 6	4 − 0 —— 4	76 + 17 —— 81	12 − 8 —— 4	1 + 8 —— 9
F	**G**	**H**	**I**	**J**
8 + 3 —— 11	76 + 6 —— 82	80 − 4 —— 84	47 − 38 —— 11	10 − 5 —— 5
K	**L**	**M**	**N**	**O**
2 + 8 —— 10	0 + 6 —— 6	57 − 9 —— 52	431 − 31 —— 400	15 + 66 —— 81

Scoring: Write in the number of digits correct and incorrect for each problem.

Problem	Digits Correct	Digits Incorrect
A		
B		
C		
D		
E		
F		
G		
H		
I		
J		
K		
L		
M		
N		
O		

Answer Key to Exercise 3

Problem	Digits Correct	Digits Incorrect
A	1	0
B	1	0
C	0	2
D	1	0
E	1	0
F	2	0
G	2	0
H	0	2
I	0	2
J	1	0
K	2	0
L	1	0
M	0	2
N	3	0
O	2	0

Comments

The results of this math probe show several things. First, the digits-correct data place the student within the instructional level for students working within second-grade materials. However, the digits-incorrect results show that the student is making too many errors to be considered instructional. Therefore, the outcome of the probe would demonstrate that the student is in the frustrational level for second-grade material. A careful examination of the probe, however, shows specifically the type of skills that the student has yet to learn. The results show that the student knows basic addition and subtraction facts. However, whenever faced with a problem in which regrouping was required, the student instead subtracted the lower from higher number. The probe suggests that the student has not yet acquired the knowledge of how to regroup in subtraction. Interestingly, the results of problems G and O indicate that the difficulties in regrouping may be specific to subtraction.

MAKE UP YOUR OWN ADDITION AND SUBTRACTION PROBLEM
EXERCISE HERE

A	B	C	D	E
F	G	H	I	J
K	L	M	N	O

Scoring: Write in the number of digits correct and incorrect for each problem.

Problem	Digits Correct	Digits Incorrect
A		
B		
C		
D		
E		
F		
G		
H		
I		
J		
K		
L		
M		
N		
O		

SCORING DIGITS CORRECT FOR MULTIPLICATION PROBLEMS

When multiplication is the skill assessed, counting digits correct can become more complicated. If the problem involves double-digit multiplication, then several digits are usually written below the answer line prior to reaching the final response. Because double-digit multiplication involves the operations of both multiplication and addition, a student could potentially make errors in two types of problems; that is, a student could multiply correctly but add incorrectly, thus getting the wrong answer. Likewise, a student could multiply incorrectly but add correctly, again reaching the wrong answer. If the student were to be given credit only for both multiplying *and* adding correctly, he/she could be penalized unduly for only performing one incorrect operation. Given that these metrics need to be sensitive to change over time, this would be inappropriate.

As a general rule of thumb, when digits correct are used in scoring multiplication, a student is given credit for the digit if the operation was performed correctly even if the answer itself is incorrect. For example, if a student asked to multiply a two-digit by two-digit problem did the following:

$$
\begin{array}{r}
75 \\
\times\ 26 \\
\hline
450 \\
150\_ \\
\hline
2850
\end{array}
$$

the problem would be scored by counting all digits correct below the answer line. There are a total of nine digits correct (indicated in bold) and two incorrect. Seven of the correct digits are the numbers 450 and 150(0), the last 0 being a place holder, and two digits are correct in the final answer. Thus, this student multiplied correctly but added incorrectly. The score suggests that the difficulties were in the addition portion of the problem, since the majority of digits would be scored for multiplication rather than addition.

In contrast, another student performing the same problem may have done the following:

$$
\begin{array}{r}
75 \\
\times\ 26 \\
\hline
435 \\
285\_ \\
\hline
3415
\end{array}
$$

This problem would be scored as having four digits correct (shown in bold): one digit (the 0 place holder) under the 1's column under the answer line, plus the three digits showing correct multiplication and addition. In this case, the student multiplied mostly incorrectly and added only partially correctly. Again, counting all digits except the placeholder incorrect would penalize the student unduly, when the real difficulty is only in multiplication—not in addition or in understanding the correct method for setting up a double-digit multiplication problem.

Exercise 4 is provided for the reader to practice scoring two- and three-digit multiplication problems.

Exercise 4

DIGITS CORRECT
FOR TWO- AND THREE-DIGIT MULTIPLICATION PROBLEMS

A		B		C		D		E	
	11		83		27		756		113
	× 13		× 48		× 34		× 8		× 59
	13		644		108		5648		1017
	11_		127_		81_				668_
	123		1914		918				7697

F		G		H		I		J	
	550		186		536		710		284
	× 66		× 59		× 91		× 92		× 67
	3300		1676		536		1420		1988
	1216_		4530		4824_		6390_		1704_
	15460		6106		48776		65320		19028

Scoring: Write in the number of digits correct and incorrect for each problem.

Problem	Digits Correct	Digits Incorrect
A		
B		
C		
D		
E		
F		
G		
H		
I		
J		

Answer Key to Exercise 4:

Problem	Digits Correct	Digits Incorrect
A	7	1
B	7	5
C	9	0
D	2	2
E	10	2
F	10	4
G	7	5
H	13	0
I	14	0
J	14	0

Comments

The results of this probe show that the student, in general, understands the procedure for conducting two- and three-digit multiplication. Errors in place value or setup of the problems are not evident. However, the student does make the mistake of operations when the second digit is supposed to be multiplied. On problems B and F, for example, the student added instead of multiplied. On problem G, the student erred in place values, which resulted in many errors. Finally, it is important to remember to give the student credit for leaving a blank (zero place holder) in the appropriate columns in most problems. It should also be noted that the when the student multiplied incorrectly, he/she sometimes added correctly. Thus, credit is given for the student's completing the operation correctly.

MAKE UP YOUR OWN MULTIPLICATION PROBLEM EXERCISE HERE

A	B	C	D	E
F	G	H	I	J

Scoring: Write in the number of digits correct and incorrect for each problem.

Problem	Digits Correct	Digits Incorrect
A		
B		
C		
D		
E		
F		
G		
H		
I		
J		

SCORING DIGITS CORRECT FOR DIVISION PROBLEMS

Division creates several unique problems in the scoring of digits correct and incorrect. Division involving two or more digits requires that students perform three operations, division, multiplication, and subtraction. If one tries to use the digits correct and incorrect metric, it quickly becomes very complex to accurately score these problems. As with multiple digit multiplication, the rule of thumb for scoring digits correct for division is that digits are counted as correct if the operation is performed correctly and the correct place value is used. For example, in the following example the student begins the long division problem correctly. (The student's work is shown on the left, the problem done entirely correctly is shown on the right)

$$
\begin{array}{r}
283 \\
25{\overline{\smash{\big)}\,7375}} \\
\underline{50} \\
237 \\
\underline{200} \\
75 \\
\underline{50} \\
25
\end{array}
\qquad\qquad
\begin{array}{r}
296 \\
25{\overline{\smash{\big)}\,7375}} \\
\underline{50} \\
237 \\
\underline{225} \\
125 \\
\underline{125} \\
0
\end{array}
$$

The student begins by dividing correctly (i.e., 73/25 = 2) and multiplies correctly (i.e., 2 × 25 = 50). He places the 50 under the correct columns and subtracts correctly (i.e., 73 – 50 = 23), and carries down the 7 from the next column. No errors have been made so far. He then makes an error in division (i.e., 237/25 = 8) but does multiply correctly (i.e., 25 × 8 = 200). He then makes an error in subtraction (i.e., 237 – 200 = 7) and carries down the 5 from the next column. He divides correctly but multiplies incorrectly (i.e., 25 × 3 = 50). Finally, he subtracts correctly. He is unsure what to do with the remainder, which, of course, is incorrect in the problem. In this problem, using the rule that correct operations are counted as correct digits, the student scores 14 digits correct (see the items in bold) and three incorrect. Looking at the type of errors provides clues as to the student's difficulties (in this case, he erred in basic division), but the scoring of the problem became complex, since many of the digits derived by the student did not match the correct solution to the problem. Furthermore, once the error in division was made, the remainder of the problem was incorrect.

A modification to the scoring procedure can reduce the problems that emerge in long division when using the rule of counting correct operations as correct. One simply compares the student's long division to a correct model of long division. The number of digits correct are summed and a percentage of correct digits out of the total digits possible for the problem is calculated.

The same example is presented below, with the student's work on the left and the model of the correct answer on the right. However, the scoring procedure used here is the percentage of correct digits. Only those digits that are in the correct place and with the correct value are counted.

```
        283                                  296
   25) 7375                             25) 7375
        50                                   50
       237                                  237
       200                                  225
        75                                  125
        50                                  125
        25                                    0
```

In the example, the student is given credit for the initial correct division (i.e., 73/25 = 2) and multiplication (i.e., 25 × 2 = 50). The student subtracted correctly (i.e., 73 − 50 = 23), brought the correct number down to the next column but began to make errors when he/she divided incorrectly (i.e., 237/25 = 8). From this point forward, the only digits that were counted as correct were the 2 and 5, which were correct compared to the model. The total number of digits that were possible in the problem were 18 (17 digits plus a zero remainder; if a student did not write the zero, he/she would be given credit for an implied digit). The student had 8 of 18 digits correct, or 44.4% of the total possible digits correct. It is strongly suggested that this method of scoring long division be used.

Exercise 5 provides opportunities to practice scoring division problems for digits correct using the method of matching the student's performance against a correct model.

DIGITS CORRECT FOR DIVISION PROBLEMS
USING THE MATCH-TO-MODEL METHOD
(CORRECT DIGITS IN SAMPLE IN BOLDFACE)

A

```
        50 R3
    14)703
        70
         3
```

B

```
        1410 R2
     3)452
        3
        15
        12
        32
        30
         2
```

C

```
        10 R4
    88)884
        88
        04
         0
         4
```

D

```
        440
    22)9950
        88
        1150
        880
         70
```

E

```
        303
    29)8787
        87
         8
         0
        87
        87
         0
```

A—Correct Model

```
        50 R3
    14)703
        70
        *3   3
         0  OR
         3
```

*0 in this position is implicit and counted as a digit correct.

B—Correct Model

```
        150 R2
     3)452
        3
        15
        15
        *2   2
         0  OR
         2
```

*0 in this position is implicit and counted as a digit correct.

C—Correct Model

```
        10 R4
    88)884
        88
        *4   4
         0  OR
         4
```

*0 in this position is implicit and counted as a digit correct.

D—Correct Model

```
        452 R6
    22)9950
        88
        115
        110
         50
         44
          6
```

E—Correct Model

```
        303
    29)8787
        87
        *8  OR  87
         0      87
        87       0
         0**
```

*0 in this position is implicit and counted as a digit correct.

**0 remainder is implicit and counted as a correct digit.

Answer Key to Exercise 5:

Problem	Actual Digits Correct	Possible Correct
A	8	8
B	5	12
C	8	8
D	6	16
E	13	13

Comments

Notice that when a remainder is present, the student is given credit for either indicating a remainder in the answer (e.g., writing "R2" in the answer) or leaving the remainder under the last subtraction. He/she is not given credit for both. The student is not given additional credit for remainders of 0. However, he/she is given credit for implied 0 digits. For example, in problem C, the student actually wrote in the 0 digit when subtracting 88 – 88. In problem A, the student did not actually write down the 0 when he/she subtracted 70 – 70; however, this digit was counted in the number of digits correct and possible for the problem. In addition, when student used appropriate short cuts, he/she was credited for all digits to solve the problem, as if he/she had not used shortcuts. Examples A, B, C, and E illustrate the use of a shortcut and the full model for completing the problem.

MAKE UP YOUR OWN DIVISION PROBLEM EXERCISE HERE

A	B	C	D	E
F	G	H	I	J
K	L	M	N	O

Scoring: Write in the number of digits correct and incorrect for each problem.

Problem	Digits Correct	Digits Incorrect
A		
B		
C		
D		
E		
F		
G		
H		
I		
J		
K		
L		
M		
N		
O		

MATH CONCEPTS–APPLICATIONS

A curriculum-based assessment of mathematics needs to go beyond math computation. The ability of children to engage in problem solving, to apply mathematical principles to problems in geometry, time, money, measurement, graphing, numeration, and other such skills, is crucial to fully identifying targets for potential intervention. Assessing student performance across time in these skills will provide strong opportunities to link the assessment and instructional process.

Several commercial products are available to help evaluators conduct a CBA for math concepts–applications. For example, Schoolhouse Technologies (*www.schoolhousetech.com*) offers sets of worksheets that cover almost every area of mathematics. These worksheets contain single-skill problems that allow in-depth assessment of each area of math applications. Other products are available from *www.edhelper.com* and *aplusmath.com* where users can build their own mixed-skills worksheet.

Another product that has been found to be very user friendly is available from Pro-Ed, Inc. (*www.proedinc.com*). Developed by Fuchs, Hamlett, and Fuchs (1999a) as part of a computerized progress monitoring system, this product contains 30 mixed-skills worksheets each for grades 2–8. The worksheets are scored by summing the number of correct answers that a student attains and dividing by the total number of possible correct problems. An example of one of these worksheets in provided in Figure 11.

Name _____ Date _____ Test 4 Page 2

Column C   Applications 4   Column D

(8)

Write the number pair that goes
With the point.

(____, ____) point A

(9)

Write the number in each blank.

$$5\overline{)13}^{\;2\;R3}$$

The quotient is _____.

The divisor is _____.

The remainder is _____.

(10)   Rewrite as a decimal.

(A) $\dfrac{6}{100}$ = _____

(A) $\dfrac{86}{100}$ = _____

(11)

There are 4 shelves for books. Each shelf holds
6 books. How many books can fit on the
bookshelves?

_____

(12)

Look at this number.
        46.9
Which digit is in the tenths place? _____

(13)

Write the number in the blank.

thirty-nine thousand, twenty-five

_____

(14)

Complete the sequence.

87,   85,   83,   ____,   ____

(15)

Write the fraction when:

8 is the denominator and
2 is numerator.

7 is the numerator and
6 is the denominator

(16)

Put these numbers in order from
the smallest to the largest in value.

67, 418   64,389   67,453

_____   _____   _____

(17)

Write >, <, or = in the blank.

$\dfrac{4}{9}$ _____ $\dfrac{5}{9}$

FIGURE 11. Example of a concepts–application probe for grade 4. From Fuchs, Hamlett, and Fuchs (1999a). Copyright 1999 by Pro-Ed, Inc. Reprinted by permission.

Spelling

USING CORRECT LETTER SEQUENCES IN SCORING SPELLING

As we have just seen, an examiner provides students with partial credit for responses in math using the digits correct metric rather than simply problems correct. An analogous metric exists for spelling—"correct letter sequences." By counting the number of correct consecutive letters rather than just the words spelled completely correctly, the examiner can detect small improvements in a student's responses. In addition, the types of errors made can be diagnostic; they can help the examiner identify the skills that a student has mastered and the ones that need to be targeted in future interventions.

Scoring correct letter sequences can be quite tedious and time-consuming. Fuchs, Fuchs, and Hamlett (1990) have devised a computer program that will provide the evaluator with automatic scoring for correct letter sequences. Although the program only works with the word lists provided by Fuchs et al., the program's output offers extensive diagnostic information for the teacher in designing instructional programs (see Figures 12 and 13). Unfortunately, the computer program is only available for the Macintosh series computers, and upgrades to more sophisticated hardware are not anticipated.

SCORING CORRECT LETTER SEQUENCES

- **Step 1:** The examiner places a blank before the first and last letter of each word to be scored. The blank is considered as a correct phantom character and is used to enable the initial and ending letters of words to be counted. For example:

```
-----------------------------------------------------------------------
    NAME: Charles Landrum          Spelling 4              Date: 4/10        Page 1
-----------------------------------------------------------------------


    Corrects       (100% LS)              14 word(s)
    Near Misses    (60-99%  LS)           19 word(s)
    Moderate Misses (10-59% LS)           16 word(s)
    Far Misses     (0-19% LS)              1 word(s)
```

Type	Correct	Possible	Pct	Type	Correct	Possible	Pct
Sing cons	48	50	96	Final vow	3	7	42
Blend	7	10	70	Double	3	4	75
FSLZ	0	0	100	c/s	0	1	0
Single vow	21	31	67	c/ck	0	2	0
Digraph	6	8	75	-le	4	7	57
Vowel + N	6	8	75	Ch/tch	2	2	100
Dual cons	13	25	52	-dge	0	1	0
Final e	1	5	52	Vowel team	4	12	33
igh/ign	0	0	100	Suffix	5	6	83
ild/old	0	0	100	tion/sion	0	1	0
a+l+cons	0	0	100	ance/ence	0	0	100
Vowel + R	9	14	64	sure/ture	0	0	100

KEY ERRORS

Dual cons	Final e	Final vow
learner—leaner	alone—alon	taste—tast
sample—samble	knife—knif	hero—hearow
chart—chard	rare—rar	lazy—lazz
mumble—mobble	cube—cub	unlucky—unluke
tractor—trater		
apart—apeot		

FIGURE 12. Example of skills analysis in spelling from Monitoring Basic Skills Progress. From Fuchs, Fuchs, Hamlett, and Allinder (1991, p. 56). Copyright 1991 by the National Association of School Psychologists. Reprinted by permission.

_ s a m p l e _

- **Step 2:** A linking symbol (⌣) is used to connect each letter to the next, beginning with the initial blank before the first letter. These should be placed alternately above and below consecutive letters.

⌣s⌣a⌢m⌣p⌢l⌣e⌢_

- **Step 3:** The examiner counts the number of letter sequences that are correct. The word *sample* above has a total of seven possible correct letter sequences.

Special Scoring Situations

Certain words create a need for special rules and conventions. In particular, the presence of double consonants can be confusing when using the letter sequences metric. If the student omits one of the consonants, credit is only given once. By comparing the student's spelling with the correct spelling, this can become evident. For example, the word

⌣b⌣u⌢b⌣b⌢l⌣e⌢ _

contains a total of seven possible letter sequences. A student who spells the word as

Spelling

NAME: Charles Landrum	Spelling D	Date: 9/1	Page 2

Corrects (100% LS)

100	March . . . . March
100	death . . . . death
100	sometimes . . . . . . sometimes
100	thankful . . . . thankful
100	baker . . . . baker
100	uncover . . . . uncover
100	shy . . . . shy
100	weakness . . . . . . weakness
100	forgot . . . . forgot
100	eyes . . . . eyes
100	army . . . . army
100	powerless . . . . . . powerless
100	wife . . . . wife
100	mix . . . . mix

Near Misses (60–99% LS)

77	shipment . . . . shapment	Single vow	
75	instead . . . . insted	Vowel team	
75	patches . . . . patces	Digraph	
75	moisten . . . . mosten	Vowel team	
75	quieter . . . . quieter	Vowel team	
75	learner . . . . learner	Dual cons	
75	trouble . . . . trubble	Vowel team	
71	sample . . . . sample	Dual cons	
71	listen . . . . lesten	Single vow	
66	badge . . . . bage	-dge	
66	taste . . . . tast	Final vow	
66	chart . . . . chard		Dual cons
66	alone . . . . alon	Final *e*	
66	restless . . . . reasless	Blend	
66	knife . . . . knif	Final *e*	
60	hero . . . . hearow	Final vow	Vowel + R
60	rare . . . . rar		Final *e*
60	cube . . . . cub	Final *e*	
60	lazy . . . . lazz	Final vow	

Moderate Misses (20–59% LS)

57	tickle . . . . teakle	C/ck	Single vow	
57	french . . . . fanch	Vowel + N	Blend	
57	mumble . . . . mobble	Dual cons	Single vow	
50	unlucky . . . . unluke	Final vow	c/ck	
50	apart . . . . apeot	Vowel + R	Dual cons	
44	calendar . . . . calendar	Vowel + R	Vowel + N	Sing cons
42	mumble . . . . mommbe	-le	Single vow	
40	rail . . . . real	Vowel team		
37	station . . . . stanch	tion/sion		
28	sample . . . . scembe	-le	Dual cons	Single vow
25	certain . . . . chanteen	Vowel team	Vowel + R	c/s
20	limb . . . . lem	Dual cons	Single vow	
20	treatment . . . . . . tempemt	Suffix	Vowel team	Blend
20	limb . . . . learn	Dual cons	Single vow	

Far Misses (0–19% LS)

| 14 | giggle . . . . gelly | -le | Double | Single vow |

FIGURE 13. Example of page 2 of a CBM skills analysis in spelling. From Fuchs, Fuchs, Hamlett, and Allinder (1991, p. 57). Copyright 1991 by the National Association of School Psychologists. Reprinted by permission.

_⌒b‿u⌒b‿l⌒e_

would be scored as having six letter sequences correct. The connection between _ and b, b and u, u and b is correct. The lack of the second b results in an incorrect sequence (no second b), but other sequences are correct.

Sample exercises for practicing scoring of spelling using correct letter sequences are provided.

Exercise 6
SCORING FOR LETTERS IN SEQUENCE FOR SPELLING

Instructions: Listed below are the actual way in which students spelled words on a weekly spelling test. The correct spelling is provided in the next column. Indicate the number of correct letter sequences for each word. The following page provides an answer sheet.

Word Spelled by Student	Correct Spelling	Letter Sequences Correct/Total Possible	Word Spelled Correctly?
rain	rain		
belong	belong		
botin	button		
lat	salt		
clock	clock		
smart	smart		
stap	step		
shep	sheep		
mint	minute		
above	above		
greup	group		
hunt	hut		
kesz	crazy		
jock	joke		
mire	mirror		
riad	drove		
nose	noise		

ANSWER SHEET FOR EXERCISE 6

Note: The first two words are scored as examples.

Word Spelled by Student	Correct Spelling	Letter Sequences Correct/Total Possible	Word Spelled Correctly?
_⌃r_a⌃i_n⌃_	rain	5/5	√
_⌃b_e⌃l_o⌃n_g⌃_	belong	7/7	√
botin	button	2/7	
slat	salt	2/5	
clock	clock	6/6	√
smart	smart	6/6	√
stap	step	3/5	
shep	sheep	4/6	
mint	minute	3/7	
above	above	6/6	√
greup	group	3/6	
hunt	hut	3/5	
kesz	crazy	0/6	
jock	joke	2/5	
mire	mirror	3/7	
riad	drove	0/6	
nose	noise	4/6	

SCORING FOR LETTERS IN SEQUENCE FOR SPELLING

Instructions: Listed below are the actual way in which students spelled words on a weekly spelling test. The correct spelling is provided in the next column. Indicate the number of correct letter sequences for each word. The following page provides an answer sheet.

Word Spelled by Student	Correct Spelling	Letter Sequences Correct/Total Possible	Word Spelled Correctly?
scad	scold		
srey	sorry		
tow	tall		
hapin	happen		
fi	fourth		
alive	alive		
give	given		
dip	drop		
terth	teeth		
beer	bear		
beck	drink		
sotp	stop		
north	north		
jell	jail		
thre	flower		
leve	leave		
insiad	inside		

ANSWER SHEET FOR EXERCISE 7

Note: The first two words are scored as examples.

Word Spelled by Student	Correct Spelling	Letter Sequences Correct/Total Possible	Word Spelled Correctly?
⌐s͜ c a d⌐	scold	3/6	
⌐s r e y⌐	sorry	2/6	
tow	tall		
hapin	happen		
fi	fourth		
alive	alive		√
give	given		
dip	drop		
terth	teeth		
beer	bear		
beck	drink		
sotp	stop		
north	north		√
jell	jail		
thre	flower		
leve	leave		
insiad	inside		

♦♦♦
Written Language
♦

Written language assessments collected as part of the assessment of academic skills problems can be scored in multiple ways. Each of these metrics is used for a somewhat different purpose.

SCORING FOR WORDS WRITTEN

The simplest metric is to count the total number of words written. This metric is a strategy commonly used when the purpose of the assessment is progress monitoring. When an evaluator is using this metric, a word is counted if it is separated from other words in the written material. Words are counted regardless of whether they are spelled correctly or are phonetically recognizable. For example, a student given the story starter "When my video game started predicting the future, I knew I had to . . . " wrote the following during a 3-minute period: "got my mom to check it out I was ckerd it was hard to recat but my mom holped me then my brather came in to my room he holped me to but he left my room want down." Notice that many of the "words" are not recognizable, nor did they make sense in the context of the story as subsequently dictated by the student. The number of words written, however, would be scored as 39.

SCORING FOR WRITING MECHANICS

When the evaluator is interested more in short-term monitoring and the development of effective interventions, strengths and weaknesses in the mechanics of writing need to be assessed. This is most easily accomplished by developing a checklist that can be used repeatedly after each written language assessment is administered. Form 8 provides an example of a quality evaluation measure that one could use for assessing mechanics such as capitalization, punctuation, sentence construction, paragraph construction, and appearance of the written product. Exercise 8 provides a set of written responses from students to practice scoring using all three sets of measures.

ASSESSING QUALITY OF LONGER WRITING SAMPLES

The evaluator may also be interested in the overall quality of the student's writing. Overall quality can be assessed by using holistic scoring metrics for longer, more elaborate assignments given as part of the instructional process. These measures usually assign scores on a scale (such as 1–5), with the criteria for each score described. Examples of two types of these scoring devices are provided in Forms 9 and 10.

Form 8

QUALITY EVALUATION MEASURE FOR WRITTEN PRODUCTS—
ELEMENTARY LEVEL

Student Name: _____

Date: _____

Grade: _____

Rating Scale:

   3 = Skill used consistently and accurately throughout written product
       (> 95% of time)

   2 = Skill used frequently and accurately throughout written product
       (50–94% of time)

   1 = Skill used infrequently or inaccurately
       (< 50% of the time)

   0 = No evidence of skill

Capitalization

First words in sentences are capitalized		0	1	2	3
Proper nouns are capitalized		0	1	2	3
Capitals are not used improperly		0	1	2	3

Punctuation

Punctuation occurs at the end of each sentence		0	1	2	3
End punctuation is correct		0	1	2	3

Sentence Construction

Absence of run-on sentences		0	1	2	3
Absence of sentence fragments		0	1	2	3
Absence of nonsensical sentences		0	1	2	3

Paragraph Construction

Each paragraph contains a topic sentence	N/A	0	1	2	3
Each sentence within a paragraph relates to the topic sentence	N/A	0	1	2	3

Appearance of Written Product

Words are legible		0	1	2	3
Spacing is appropriate between letters/words		0	1	2	3
Margins are appropriate		0	1	2	3
Written product is neat, with correct spelling		0	1	2	3

TOTAL SCORE _____

Form 9

CRITERIA FOR HOLISTIC WRITING ASSESSMENT*

① Highly flawed—Not competent

- Ideas poorly communicated

- Frequent usage errors (such as agreement, pronoun misuse, tense)

- Incorrect or erratic use of capitalization, punctuation, and spelling conventions

- Sentence fragments and run-ons; few complete sentences

- No concept of paragraph construction

② Unacceptable—Not competent

- Poor organization of ideas

- Frequent usage errors (such as agreement, pronoun misuse, tense)

- Inconsistent use of capitalization, punctuation, and spelling conventions

- Sentence fragments and run-ons; few complete sentences

- Poor topic sentence; flawed paragraph development

③ Minimally competent—Acceptable

- Ideas sufficiently organized and communicated

- Only occasional usage errors (such as agreement, pronoun misuse, tense)

- Minimal number of sentence errors (fragments or run-ons)

- Paragraphs have topic sentences, supporting ideas, and closing sentences

- Some attempt at paragraph transition

④ Competent—Clear mastery

- Ideas clearly communicated and of a fairly mature quality

- No usage errors

- Correct capitalization, punctuation, and spelling

- No fragments or run-ons

- Effective paragraph construction

Note: A paper that is illegible, off the point, or a nonresponse is scored 0.

Source: Division of Curriculum and Instruction, Department of Elementary and Secondary Education, Milwaukee, Wisconsin, Public Schools.

Form 10

CRITERIA FOR ANALYTICAL SCORING*

	1	2	3	4	5	
Organization	Little or nothing is written. The essay is disorganized, incoherent, and poorly developed. The essay does not stay on the topic.		The essay is not complete. It lacks an introduction, well-developed body, or conclusion. The coherence and sequence are attempted but not adequate.		The essay is well organized. It contains an introductory, supporting, and concluding paragraph. The essay is coherent, ordered logically, and fully developed.	×6
Sentence Structure	The student writes frequent run-ons or fragments.		The student makes occasional errors in sentence structure. Little variety in sentence length or structure exists.		The sentences are complete and varied in length and structure.	×5
Usage	The student makes frequent errors in word choice and agreement.		The student makes occasional errors in word choice or agreement.		The usage is correct. Word choice is appropriate.	×4
Mechanics	The student makes frequent errors in spelling, punctuation, and capitalization.		The student makes an occasional error in mechanics.		The spelling, capitalization, and punctuation are correct.	×4
Format	The format is sloppy. There are no margins or indentations. Handwriting is inconsistent.		The handwriting, margins, and indentations have occasional inconsistencies— no title or inappropriate title.		The format is correct. The title is appropriate. The handwriting, margins, and indentations are consistent.	×1

*Source: Adams County School District #12, 11285 Highline Drive, Northglenn, Colorado 80203.

SCORING BRIEF WRITTEN LANGUAGE SAMPLES: EXAMPLES AND EXERCISES

Below are three written samples, collected as 3-minute story starters during a direct assessment of written expression. All students were in the fifth grade. In the following exercises, readers can practice using the Quality Evaluation Measure for Written Products—Elementary Level to score the samples. A scored form follows each blank form (answers are underlined).

Starter and Writing Samples

Starter: "When my video game started predicting the future, I knew I had to . . . "

Student 1: Bryan

"got my mom to check it out I was ckerd it was hard to recat but my mom holped me then my brother came in to my room he helped my to but he left my room want down."

Student 2: Valesa

"Get it to put back on my other game and when the future came on my board I was very surprised because it was talking to me and I did not now wat it was talking about and it just kep on talking to me and when it said I was going to live in mars I said y must I live on mars he said because you have to and I said how comes."

Student 3: Cary

"run and get my camera. I ran into my room to find it, it was gone. I wanted to see what it would do if I turned it off. I put my hand on the power button, and I felt a stinging shock on my finger. I ran to get my mom. By the time she got there, it was too late."

Exercise 8: Blank Form for Bryan

QUALITY EVALUATION MEASURE FOR WRITTEN PRODUCTS— ELEMENTARY LEVEL

Student Name: _____

Date: _____

Grade: _____

Rating Scale:

3 = Skill used consistently and accurately throughout written product (> 95% of time)

2 = Skill used frequently and accurately throughout written product (50–94% of time)

1 = Skill used infrequently or inaccurately (< 50% of the time)

0 = No evidence of skill

Capitalization
First words in sentences are capitalized	0	1	2	3
Proper nouns are capitalized	0	1	2	3
Capitals are not used improperly	0	1	2	3

Punctuation
Punctuation occurs at the end of each sentence	0	1	2	3
End punctuation is correct	0	1	2	3

Sentence Construction
Absence of run-on sentences	0	1	2	3
Absence of sentence fragments	0	1	2	3
Absence of nonsensical sentences	0	1	2	3

Paragraph Construction
Each paragraph contains a topic sentence	N/A	0	1	2	3
Each sentence within a paragraph relates to the topic sentence	N/A	0	1	2	3

Appearance of Written Product
Words are legible	N/A	0	1	2	3
Spacing is appropriate between letters/words	N/A	0	1	2	3
Margins are appropriate	N/A	0	1	2	3
Written product is neat, with correct spelling	N/A	0	1	2	3

TOTAL SCORE _____

Exercise 8: Scored Form for Bryan

QUALITY EVALUATION MEASURE FOR WRITTEN PRODUCTS—
ELEMENTARY LEVEL

Student Name: _Bryan_

Date: _4-21-03_

Grade: _5_

Rating Scale:

3 = Skill used consistently and accurately throughout written product (> 95% of time)

2 = Skill used frequently and accurately throughout written product (50–94% of time)

1 = Skill used infrequently or inaccurately (< 50% of the time)

0 = No evidence of skill

Capitalization

First words in sentences are capitalized	<u>0</u>	1	2	3
Proper nouns are capitalized	<u>0</u>	1	2	3
Capitals are not used improperly	<u>0</u>	1	2	3

Punctuation

Punctuation occurs at the end of each sentence	<u>0</u>	1	2	3
End punctuation is correct	<u>0</u>	1	2	3

Sentence Construction

Absence of run-on sentences	<u>0</u>	1	2	3
Absence of sentence fragments	0	<u>1</u>	2	3
Absence of nonsensical sentences	0	1	2	<u>3</u>

Paragraph Construction

Each paragraph contains a topic sentence	<u>N/A</u>	0	1	2	3
Each sentence within a paragraph relates to the topic sentence	<u>N/A</u>	0	1	2	3

Appearance of Written Product

Words are legible	<u>N/A</u>	0	1	2	3
Spacing is appropriate between letters/words	<u>N/A</u>	0	1	2	3
Margins are appropriate	<u>N/A</u>	0	1	2	3
Written product is neat, with correct spelling	<u>N/A</u>	0	1	2	3

TOTAL SCORE   _4_

Exercise 9: Blank Form for Valesa

QUALITY EVALUATION MEASURE FOR WRITTEN PRODUCTS—
ELEMENTARY LEVEL

Student Name: _____

Date: _____

Grade: _____

Rating Scale:

3 = Skill used consistently and accurately throughout written product
(> 95% of time)

2 = Skill used frequently and accurately throughout written product
(50–94% of time)

1 = Skill used infrequently or inaccurately
(< 50% of the time)

0 = No evidence of skill

Capitalization
First words in sentences are capitalized	0	1	2	3
Proper nouns are capitalized	0	1	2	3
Capitals are not used improperly	0	1	2	3

Punctuation
Punctuation occurs at the end of each sentence	0	1	2	3
End punctuation is correct	0	1	2	3

Sentence Construction
Absence of run-on sentences	0	1	2	3
Absence of sentence fragments	0	1	2	3
Absence of nonsensical sentences	0	1	2	3

Paragraph Construction
Each paragraph contains a topic sentence	N/A	0	1	2	3
Each sentence within a paragraph relates to the topic sentence	N/A	0	1	2	3

Appearance of Written Product
Words are legible	N/A	0	1	2	3
Spacing is appropriate between letters/words	N/A	0	1	2	3
Margins are appropriate	N/A	0	1	2	3
Written product is neat, with correct spelling	N/A	0	1	2	3

TOTAL SCORE _____

QUALITY EVALUATION MEASURE FOR WRITTEN PRODUCTS—
ELEMENTARY LEVEL

Student Name: _Valesa_

Date: _4-21-03_

Grade: _5_

Rating Scale:

3 = Skill used consistently and accurately throughout written product (> 95% of time)

2 = Skill used frequently and accurately throughout written product (50–94% of time)

1 = Skill used infrequently or inaccurately (< 50% of the time)

0 = No evidence of skill

Capitalization

First words in sentences are capitalized	0	<u>1</u>	2	3
Proper nouns are capitalized	0	1	<u>2</u>	3
Capitals are not used improperly	0	1	2	<u>3</u>

Punctuation

Punctuation occurs at the end of each sentence	<u>0</u>	1	2	3
End punctuation is correct	<u>0</u>	1	2	3

Sentence Construction

Absence of run-on sentences	0	1	2	<u>3</u>
Absence of sentence fragments	0	1	2	<u>3</u>
Absence of nonsensical sentences	0	1	2	<u>3</u>

Paragraph Construction

Each paragraph contains a topic sentence	N/A	0	1	2	3
Each sentence within a paragraph relates to the topic sentence	N/A	0	1	2	3

Appearance of Written Product

Words are legible	N/A	0	1	2	3
Spacing is appropriate between letters/words	N/A	0	1	2	3
Margins are appropriate	N/A	0	1	2	3
Written product is neat, with correct spelling	N/A	0	1	2	3

TOTAL SCORE _15_

QUALITY EVALUATION MEASURE FOR WRITTEN PRODUCTS—
ELEMENTARY LEVEL

Student Name: _____

Date: _____

Grade: _____

Rating Scale:

3 = Skill used consistently and accurately throughout written product
(> 95% of time)

2 = Skill used frequently and accurately throughout written product
(50–94% of time)

1 = Skill used infrequently or inaccurately
(< 50% of the time)

0 = No evidence of skill

Capitalization

First words in sentences are capitalized	0	1	2	3
Proper nouns are capitalized	0	1	2	3
Capitals are not used improperly	0	1	2	3

Punctuation

Punctuation occurs at the end of each sentence	0	1	2	3
End punctuation is correct	0	1	2	3

Sentence Construction

Absence of run-on sentences	0	1	2	3
Absence of sentence fragments	0	1	2	3
Absence of nonsensical sentences	0	1	2	3

Paragraph Construction

Each paragraph contains a topic sentence	N/A	0	1	2	3
Each sentence within a paragraph relates to the topic sentence	N/A	0	1	2	3

Appearance of Written Product

Words are legible	N/A	0	1	2	3
Spacing is appropriate between letters/words	N/A	0	1	2	3
Margins are appropriate	N/A	0	1	2	3
Written product is neat, with correct spelling	N/A	0	1	2	3

TOTAL SCORE _____

Exercise 10: Scored Form for Cary

QUALITY EVALUATION MEASURE FOR WRITTEN PRODUCTS— ELEMENTARY LEVEL

Student Name: _Cary_

Date: _4-21-03_

Grade: _5_

Rating Scale:

3 = Skill used consistently and accurately throughout written product (> 95% of time)

2 = Skill used frequently and accurately throughout written product (50–94% of time)

1 = Skill used infrequently or inaccurately (< 50% of the time)

0 = No evidence of skill

Capitalization

First words in sentences are capitalized	0	1	2	**3**
Proper nouns are capitalized	0	1	2	3
Capitals are not used improperly	0	1	2	3

Punctuation

Punctuation occurs at the end of each sentence	0	1	2	3
End punctuation is correct	0	1	2	3

Sentence Construction

Absence of run-on sentences	0	1	2	3
Absence of sentence fragments	0	1	2	3
Absence of nonsensical sentences	0	1	2	3

Paragraph Construction

Each paragraph contains a topic sentence	N/A	0	1	2	3
Each sentence within a paragraph relates to the topic sentence	N/A	0	1	2	3

Appearance of Written Product

Words are legible	N/A	0	1	2	3
Spacing is appropriate between letters/words	N/A	0	1	2	3
Margins are appropriate	N/A	0	1	2	3
Written product is neat, with correct spelling	N/A	0	1	2	3

TOTAL SCORE   _24_

♦ ♦ ♦

Summary Form
for Academic Assessment

♦

Data obtained during Steps 1 and 2 represent the collection of extensive information about a student's present level of academic performance. The data also provide a means of examining the academic environment in which the student's problems are occurring. To facilitate the process of assembling these data, a form for summarizing these data is provided.

Form 11

DATA SUMMARY FORM FOR ACADEMIC ASSESSMENT

Child's name: _____

Teacher: _____

Grade: _____

School: _____

School district: _____

Date: _____

READING—SKILLS

Primary type of reading series used

☐ Basal reader

☐ Literature-based

☐ Trade books

Secondary type of reading materials used

☐ Basal reader

☐ Literature-based

☐ Trade books

☐ None

Title of curriculum series: _____

Level/book—target student: _____

Level/book—average student: _____

Results of passages administered:

Grade level/ book	Location in book	WC/ min	Words incorrect/ min	% correct	Median scores for level			Learning level (M, I, F)
					WC	ER	%C	
	Beginning							
	Middle							
	End							
	Beginning							
	Middle							
	End							
	Beginning							
	Middle							
	End							
	Beginning							
	Middle							
	End							

READING—ENVIRONMENT

Instructional Procedures:

Primary type of reading instruction:

☐ Basal readers   ☐ Whole-language

☐ Other (describe) _____

Number of reading groups: _____

Student's reading group (if applicable): _____

Allotted time/day for reading: _____

Contingencies: _____

Teaching procedures: _____

_____

_____

Observations: _____ None completed for this area

System used:

   ☐ BOSS

   ☐ Other _____

Setting of observations:

☐ ISW:TPsnt   ☐ SmGp:Tled   ☐ Coop

☐ ISW:TSmGp   ☐ LgGp:Tled   ☐ Other _____

BOSS results:

Target	Peer	Target	Peer
AET% _____	AET% _____	OFT-M% _____	OFT-M% _____
PET% _____	PET% _____	OFT-V% _____	OFT-V% _____
		OFT-P% _____	OFT-P% _____
	TDI% _____		

Intervention Strategies Attempted:

_____ Simple _____

_____

_____ Moderate _____

_____

_____ Intensive _____

_____

TEACHER-REPORTED STUDENT BEHAVIOR

Rate the following areas from 1 to 5 (1 = very unsatisfactory, 3 = satisfactory, 5 = superior)

Reading Group

a. Oral reading ability (as evidenced in reading group) _____
b. Volunteers answers _____
c. When called upon, gives correct answer _____
d. Attends to other students when they read aloud _____
e. Knows the appropriate place in book _____

Independent Seatwork

a. Stays on task _____
b. Completes assigned work in required time _____
c. Work is accurate _____
d. Works quietly _____
e. Remains in seat when required _____

Homework (if any)

a. Handed in on time _____
b. Is complete _____
c. Is accurate _____

STUDENT-REPORTED BEHAVIOR   _____ None completed for this area

Understands expectations of teacher	☐ Yes	☐ No	☐ Not sure
Understands assignments	☐ Yes	☐ No	☐ Not sure
Feels he/she can do the assignments	☐ Yes	☐ No	☐ Not sure
Likes the subject	☐ Yes	☐ No	☐ Not sure
Feels he/she is given enough time to complete assignments	☐ Yes	☐ No	☐ Not sure
Feels like he/she is called upon to participate in discussions	☐ Yes	☐ No	☐ Not sure

MATH—SKILLS

Curriculum series used: _____

Specific problems in math: _____

Mastery skill of target student: _____

Mastery skill of average student: _____

Instructional skill of target student: _____

Instructional skill of average student: _____

Problems in math applications: _____

Results of math probes:

Probe type	No.	Digits correct/min	Digits incorrect/min	% problems correct	Learning level (M, I, F)

MATH—ENVIRONMENT
Instructional Procedures:

Number of math groups: _____

Student's group (high, middle, low): _____

Allotted time/day: _____

Teaching procedures: _____

_____

Contingencies: _____

Observations: _____ None completed for this area

System used:

    ☐ BOSS

    ☐ Other _____

Setting of observations:

☐ ISW:TPsnt   ☐ SmGp:Tled   ☐ Coop

☐ ISW:TSmGp   ☐ LgGp:Tled   ☐ Other _____

BOSS results:

Target	Peer	Target	Peer
AET% _____	AET% _____	OFT-M% _____	OFT-M% _____
PET% _____	PET% _____	OFT-V% _____	OFT-V% _____
		OFT-P% _____	OFT-P% _____
	TDI% _____		

Intervention Strategies Attempted:

_____ Simple _____

_____

_____ Moderate _____

_____

_____ Intensive _____

_____

TEACHER-REPORTED STUDENT BEHAVIOR

Rate the following areas from 1 to 5 (1 = very unsatisfactory, 3 = satisfactory, 5 = superior)

Math group (large)

a. Volunteers answers
b. When called upon, gives correct answer   _____
c. Attends to other students when they give answers   _____
d. Knows the appropriate place in math book   _____

Math Group (small)

a. Volunteers answers   _____
b. When called upon, gives correct answer   _____
c. Attends to other students when they give answers   _____
d. Knows the appropriate place in math book   _____

Math Group (cooperative)

a. Volunteers answers   _____
b. Contributes to group objectives   _____
c. Attends to other students when they give answers   _____
d. Facilitates others in group to participate   _____
e. Shows appropriate social skills in group   _____

Independent Seatwork

a. Stays on task   _____
b. Completes assigned work in required time   _____
c. Work is accurate   _____
d. Works from initial directions   _____
e. Works quietly   _____
f. Remains in seat when required   _____

Homework (if any)

a. Handed in on time   _____
b. Is complete   _____
c. Is accurate   _____

STUDENT-REPORTED BEHAVIOR ____ None completed for this area

Understands expectations of teacher	☐ Yes	☐ No	☐ Not sure
Understands assignments	☐ Yes	☐ No	☐ Not sure
Feels he/she can do the assignments	☐ Yes	☐ No	☐ Not sure
Likes the subject	☐ Yes	☐ No	☐ Not sure
Feels he/she is given enough time to complete assignments	☐ Yes	☐ No	☐ Not sure
Feels like he/she is called upon to participate in discussions	☐ Yes	☐ No	☐ Not sure

SPELLING—SKILLS

Type of material used for spelling instruction:

☐ Published spelling series

Title of series _____

☐ Basal reading series

Title of series _____

☐ Teacher-made materials

☐ Other _____

Curriculum series (if applicable): _____

Results of spelling probes:

Grade level of probe	Probe no.	LSC	% words correct	Median LSC for grade level	Level (M, I, F)
	1				
	2				
	3				
	1				
	2				
	3				
	1				
	2				
	3				
	1				
	2				
	3				

SPELLING—ENVIRONMENT

Instructional Procedures:

Allotted time/day: _____

Teaching procedures: _____

Contingencies: _____

Observations: _____ None completed for this area

System used:

□ BOSS

□ Other _____

Setting of observations:

□ ISW:TPsnt   □ SmGp:Tled   □ Coop

□ ISW:TSmGp   □ LgGp:Tled   □ Other _____

BOSS results:

Target	Peer	Target	Peer
AET% _____	AET% _____	OFT-M% _____	OFT-M% _____
PET% _____	PET% _____	OFT-V% _____	OFT-V% _____
		OFT-P% _____	OFT-P% _____
	TDI% _____		

Intervention Strategies Attempted:

_____ Simple _____

_____

_____ Moderate _____

_____

_____ Intensive _____

_____

STUDENT-REPORTED BEHAVIOR   _____ None completed for this area

Understands expectations of teacher	□ Yes	□ No	□ Not sure
Understands assignments	□ Yes	□ No	□ Not sure
Feels he/she can do the assignments	□ Yes	□ No	□ Not sure
Likes the subject	□ Yes	□ No	□ Not sure
Feels he/she is given enough time to complete assignments	□ Yes	□ No	□ Not sure
Feels like he/she is called upon to participate in discussions	□ Yes	□ No	□ Not sure

WRITING—SKILLS

Types of writing assignments: _____

Areas of difficulty:

Content:

☐ Expressing thoughts

☐ Story length

☐ Story depth

☐ Creativity

Mechanics:

☐ Capitalization

☐ Punctuation

☐ Grammar

☐ Handwriting

☐ Spelling

Results of written expression probes:

Story starter	Words written	Instructional level?	Comments

WRITING—ENVIRONMENT

Instructional Procedures:

Allotted time/day: _____

Teaching procedures: _____

_____

Observations: _____ None completed for this area

System used:

   ☐ BOSS

   ☐ Other _____

Setting of observations:

☐ ISW:TPsnt   ☐ SmGp:Tled   ☐ Coop

☐ ISW:TSmGp   ☐ LgGp:Tled   ☐ Other _____

BOSS results:

Target	Peer	Target	Peer
AET% _____	AET% _____	OFT-M% _____	OFT-M% _____
PET% _____	PET% _____	OFT-V% _____	OFT-V% _____
		OFT-P% _____	OFT-P% _____
	TDI% _____		

STUDENT-REPORTED BEHAVIOR   _____ None completed for this area

Understands expectations of teacher	☐ Yes	☐ No	☐ Not sure
Understands assignments	☐ Yes	☐ No	☐ Not sure
Feels he/she can do the assignments	☐ Yes	☐ No	☐ Not sure
Likes the subject	☐ Yes	☐ No	☐ Not sure
Feels he/she is given enough time to complete assignments	☐ Yes	☐ No	☐ Not sure
Feels like he/she is called upon to participate in discussions	☐ Yes	☐ No	☐ Not sure

STEP 3

◆ ◆ ◆

Instructional Modification

◆

◆ ◆ ◆
The Folding-In Technique
◆

The "folding-in" technique has been found to be a powerful and easy-to-implement strategy that can be useful in any intervention whose objective is for a student to acquire new, fact-based information. The intervention can cut across subjects and can be used for anything from teaching students letter recognition in kindergarten, to word recognition, to multiplication facts, to events leading up to the Civil War, to chemical formulas.

Based upon the suggested ratios of Gickling's model of curriculum-based assessment (Gickling & Havertape, 1981), the procedure attempts to build success and momentum for acquisition of new information. By assessing a student's entry knowledge of the skill to be learned, the evaluator can determine the material a student already knows and the material that is unknown. When the new material is taught, the ratio of known to unknown material is maintained at no greater than 70% known and 30% unknown. Thus, a student who is being exposed to new material is never asked to try to learn more than 30% of what is presented.

The folding-in technique is based in part upon findings about the amount of repetition a student needs in order to master new information (Hargis, Terhaar-Yonkers, Williams, & Reed, 1988). Learning is conceptualized as a process described in Figure 14. In the acquisition stage, a student begins to be exposed to new material; in the mastery stage, the student becomes fluent with the material; and in the generalization and adaptation stages, the student discovers ways of applying the same or similar knowledge to novel situations. At an IQ level of 100, it takes approximately 35 repetitions for material to move from a level of acquisition to mastery. As the IQ goes up to 115, the number of repetitions decreases to about 15. At an IQ of 85, the number of repetitions increases to about 55 (Burns, 2001; MacQuarrie, Tucker, Burns, & Hartman, 2002). The folding-in technique is

Level	Emphasis	Strategies
Acquisition	Achieving accurate responding	Demonstration, modeling, cues, prompting
Mastery	Accuracy with speed	Routine and novel drill and practice
Generalization	Performance and response under novel stimuli	Training discrimination and differentiation
Adaptation	Performance of similar responses under novel stimuli	Problem solving, role playing, training under simulation conditions

FIGURE 14. Stages of the learning process.

designed to maximize the number of repetitions to new material within a short period of time, thereby facilitating the student's progress from the acquisition to the mastery level of learning.

To illustrate the technique, it is described in detail for use in teaching word recognition and reading fluency, and acquisition of multiplication facts within a peer-tutoring context. Again, it is important for the reader to recognize that the technique can be applied to any content area where fact-based knowledge needs to be learned.

EXAMPLE: FOLDING-IN TECHNIQUE FOR WORD ACQUISITION AND READING FLUENCY

• **Step 1:** The evaluator selects a passage for the student to read. The passage should be one that the student is currently working on in class. It is important that the passage contain no more than 50% unknown material. This can be assessed by conducted a word search. The evaluator simply asks the student to read and explain the meaning of various key words from the passage. If the student misses more than 50% of the words in the word search, the evaluator should select a different passage and repeat the process.

• **Step 2:** The evaluator asks the student to read a portion of the passage (usually a paragraph or two) aloud and times the reading. The evaluator marks the point in the passage reached by the student at the end of 1 minute. The number of words read correctly in this minute is designated as the presession reading fluency.

• **Step 3:** As the student reads, the evaluator notes at least three words that the student has difficulty with or doesn't seem to understand. On 3″ × 5″ index cards, the evaluator writes the three words (one on each card). These words are designated as "unknowns." If more than three words can be designated as unknown, the evaluator selects words that are meaningful and help the student to understand the story.

• **Step 4:** On 3″ × 5″ index cards, the evaluator writes seven words (one on each card) from the passage that the student does seem to know. These should be words that are meaningful to the passage, not simply *and, the,* or other non-meaningful expressions.

- **Step 5:** The session begins with presentation of the first unknown word. The evaluator should define the word for the student and use it in a sentence. Next, the evaluator should ask the student to repeat the definition and use it in a different sentence.

- **Step 6:** Now the folding-in begins. After the unknown word is presented, one of the known words is presented. The student is asked to say the word aloud. Next, the unknown word is again presented, followed by the known word previously presented, and then a new known word. This sequence of presentation (unknown followed by knowns) is continued until all seven knowns and the one unknown word have been presented.

Next, the second unknown word is presented in the same way as the first, with the evaluator and then the student defining it and using it in a sentence. This second unknown word is then folded in among the other seven known words and the one unknown word. In the course of the multiple presentations of the words, the student is asked to repeat the unknown word's definition and to use it in a sentence whenever he/she hesitates or is incorrect in the pronunciation of the word. Finally, the third unknown is folded in among the other nine words (two unknown, seven known). Given that the other words were assessed to be known at the starting point, the student should not have any difficulty with these words. Figure 15 illustrates the full sequence of presentations for a set of 10 words.

- **Step 7:** Upon completion of the folding-in intervention, the student is asked to reread the passage. The evaluator again marks the number of seconds it took for the student to reach the point in the passage reached at 1 minute during the presession reading. It is important that the student read at least to the same point of the passage that he/she reached at the beginning of the session; this is necessary to establish accuracy in the oral reading rate measure. The score obtained here is considered the student's postsession reading score.

- **Step 8:** Both the pre- and postsession scores are graphed (usually by the student). These data can be very useful in showing the student the consistent improvement in his/her reading skills over the short period of time in each session, as well as the acquisition of material over days and weeks.

- **Step 9:** The next session begins by having the student read the next portion of the passage. Following the reading, the 10 words (seven known, three unknown) that were used in the previous session are reviewed. A mark is placed on one of the unknown words to designate that the student knew the word without hesitation during this session.

- **Step 10:** A criterion is set to determine when a previously unknown word is designated as a known word. Typically, this may be defined as getting the word correct on two consecutive sessions after it was introduced.

- **Step 11:** As a new unknown word is added to the drill procedure, one of the original known words is removed from the pile. The first word to be removed is one of the original known words selected on the first session. Each of the other seven known words are replaced with new unknown words. Finally, by the time one of the original unknown words is removed from the pile, it will have been drilled far in excess of the required 55 repetitions for new material to reach mastery levels.

EXAMPLE: FOLDING-IN TECHNIQUE
FOR MULTIPLICATION FACTS

Students: Two boys in third-grade special education class. Both boys referred for problems in learning multiplication facts.

Preassessment Phase: To determine the number of known and unknown facts, the students are administered a quiz in which they are asked to answer all computational problems with fact families 1–9. The number of problems not completed or incorrect provides an indication of the facts that have and have not been learned.

Instructional Structure: The procedure is set up as a peer-tutoring activity. The students are taught the procedure and are required to conduct 10-minute tutoring sessions in which they drill each other using the folding-in technique.

- **Step 1:** Each student selects seven cards from their pile of preassessed known facts.
- **Step 2:** Each student selects one card from their unknown pile of preassessed facts.
- **Step 3:** The two students are informed by the teacher that they have 20 minutes to begin tutoring.
- **Step 4:** After it is decided which student will begin the tutoring, the folding-in procedure begins. The teacher of the pair presents the first unknown fact to the learner. The learner is required to write the fact on a piece of paper, say it to him-/herself three times, and then turn the paper over.
- **Step 5:** The teacher than presents a known fact, followed by the unknown fact, the first known fact, and another known fact. The unknown fact is presented sequentially in this fashion until all seven known facts have been presented and folded-in among the unknown facts. (See Figure 15 for presentation sequence.)
- **Step 6:** The group of eight facts (one unknown and seven known) are shuffled. The second unknown fact is then presented and folded-in among the other eight facts. This is repeated again for the third unknown fact.
- **Step 7:** If the student hesitates or is incorrect on any fact, the teacher instructs him/her to complete a brief correction procedure. The teacher tells him/her the correct answer and has him/her write the incorrect fact three times. The incorrect fact is then presented again to the learner.
- **Step 8:** When all facts have been folded in, the entire group of 10 facts is presented three times. Each time, the packet of index cards is shuffled to prevent the learner from simply remembering the sequence of responses.
- **Step 9:** The final step is a test of the 10 facts that the students have practiced. On this test, a mark is placed on the unknown fact cards if a student is correct on this trial. When an unknown fact attains three consecutive marks, it is considered as a learned fact.
- **Step 10:** The number of new facts learned each week is graphed by the students. In addition, the teacher administers weekly curriculum-based measurement math probes taken from across all fact families. These data are also graphed.

Presentation no.	Unknown item no.	Known item no.	Presentation no.	Unknown item no.	Known item no.	Presentation no.	Unknown item no.	Known item no.
1	1		42		2	83	3	
2		1	43		3	84	2	
3	1		44	2		85	1	
4		1	45	1		86		1
5		2	46		1	87		2
6	1		47		2	88		3
7		1	48		3	89	3	
8		2	49		4	90	2	
9		3	50	2		91	1	
10	1		51	1		92		1
11		1	52		1	93		2
12		2	53		2	94		3
13		3	54		3	95		4
14		4	55		4	96	3	
15	1		56		5	97	2	
16		1	57	2		98	1	
17		2	58	1		99		1
18		3	59		1	100		2
19		4	60		2	101		3
20		5	61		3	102		4
21	1		62		4	103		5
22		1	63		5	104	3	
23		2	64		6	105	2	
24		3	65	2		106	1	
25		4	66	1		107		1
26		5	67		1	108		2
27		6	68		2	109		3
28	1		69		3	110		4
29		1	70		4	111		5
30		2	71		5	112		6
31		3	72		6	113	3	
32		4	73		7	114	2	
33		5	74	3		115	1	
34		6	75	2		116		1
35		7	76	1		117		2
36	2		77		1	118		3
37	1		78	3		119		4
38		1	79	2		120		5
39	2		80	1		121		6
40	1		81		1	122		7
41		1	82		2			

FIGURE 15. Sequences for presenting known and unknown materials in the folding-in technique, assuming 10 items (3 unknown and 7 known).

STEP 4

♦♦♦

Progress Monitoring

♦

♦ ♦ ♦

Graphing Data

♦

One of the key components of progress monitoring is providing a visual display of the outcomes of the data collection process. Such graphic displays serve to improve the evaluator's own understanding of the data; they also offer an effective mechanism for communicating with parents, teachers, and students themselves about the student progress. Indeed, the process of collecting and reporting the data in a graphic form can itself serve as a strong motivator and reinforcer for some students.

Provided below are instructions for setting up hand-drawn graphs. However, evaluators should consider the use of existing graphing tools to display and manage the data. Spreadsheet programs such as Microsoft EXCEL, Quatro-Pro, or Delta Graph are all common tools that can easily be developed for graphing purposes. In addition, AIMSweb (*www.aimsweb.com*) offers an excellent commercial product that is specifically designed to collect, manage, and display progress monitoring data.

SETTING UP GRAPHIC DISPLAYS

Graphic displays of data are useful for both short- and long-term monitoring. The setting-up process is similar for all types of graphs.

• **Step 1:** Identify the metric that is being used for data collection purposes. This can be words correct or incorrect per minute, cumulative problems learned, number of pages mastered, number of homework problems done correctly, or other such measures.

• **Step 2:** Identify the possible range that the metric used for data collection can occupy. This can be any set of numbers representing the lower and upper limits that the measure is likely to attain.

• **Step 3:** The metric used for data collection becomes the range placed on the *y* (vertical) axis. Divide the range into equal units, and write these along the vertical axis.

• **Step 4:** Identify the amount of time across which the data will be collected. This can be any unit of time up to a full school year.

• **Step 5:** The amount of time for data collection becomes the range placed on the *x* (horizontal) axis. Divide the range into equal units (sessions, days, weeks, months, etc.).

The data are plotted by placing points on the graph, each of which indicates the outcome on the measure used for monitoring at each point in time when data are collected.

Graphs are usually divided by the particular phase of the intervention. Data obtained during baseline and intervention phases are separated by a solid line drawn on the graph. The data are also not connected by lines across these two phases. Once the intervention begins, changes in the intervention procedure are designated by broken lines, with the data again not being connected through those phases.

Figure 16 shows a graphic display for a first-grade student for whom two interventions, peer-tutoring and peer-tutoring plus curriculum-based measurement (CBM) feedback, were implemented to improve performance on acquisition of basic math facts in addition and subtraction. The intervention operated for 15 weeks (one semester). Baseline and intervention phases are separated by a solid line, and the two intervention phases are separated by a broken line.

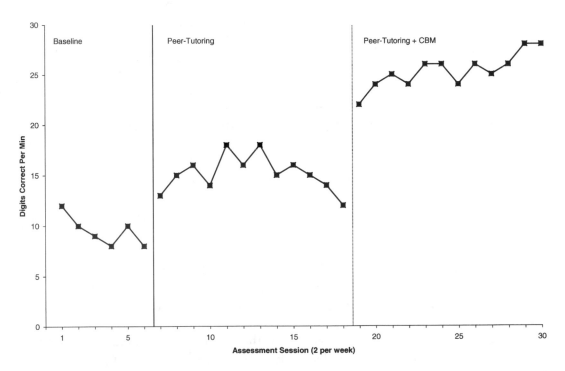

FIGURE 16. Example of reading data for a first-grade student for whom peer-tutoring and peer-tutoring plus CBM were used as interventions.

INTERPRETING GRAPHIC DATA

Deciding whether the data collected over time indicate that outcomes are moving in the expected direction can be done in several ways. Two of the most common methods of trend analysis are the quarter-intersect or split-middle method of White and Haring (1980), or the more mathematically precise method of calculating an ordinary least squares (OLS) trend line.

Quarter-Intersect (or Split-Middle) Method

To illustrate the first method of trend estimation, a step-by-step example is provided.

Figure 17A displays the data from the peer-tutoring phase (see Figure 16) of the intervention program described earlier, designed to improve the math computation performance of a first-grade student. To calculate a trend estimation, the following is done:

- **Step 1:** Divide the entire data series of interest into two equal parts. If the number of data points is odd, then the middle data point of the series becomes the dividing line. If the number of data points is even, than the data series is split between the two middle points of the data series. In this example, there are 16 data points, so the series is split between the eighth and ninth data points of the series. (See Figure 17B).
- **Step 2:** Find the median score for each of the two sets of the data series. The median score is the middle or central score among the data points. If the middle score falls between two data points, then the median score is the halfway point between these two scores. In this example, there are eight data points in each half of the series. An examination of the data in the left half of the series shows that the score of 15.5 is the median score. The score for the right half of the data series is 15.5. (See Figure 17C).
- **Step 3:** Connect the median scores for each half of the data series. (See Figure 17D). This line represents the trend estimation for the data series.

Ordinary Least Squares Method

The OLS method is the generation of a regression of the data points to a line that best fits the data series. Although OLS can be mathematically complex to calculate, the use of computers makes this measure simple to generate. Almost all graphic software products such as Microsoft EXCEL, Quarto-Pro, or Delta Graph contain a function within the program that will allow the OLS to be calculated. If one does not have access to these programs, the calculation of OLS can become problematic.

In practice, it is recommended that the OLS be used if it can be obtained, since research has shown it to be more accurate than other trend line estimation methods, such as the quarter-intersect method. Figure 18 shows the results of the OLS calculated for the same data set as that used for the quarter-intersect method in Figure 17D.

FIGURE 17. Illustration of the quarter-intersect or split-middle method of trend estimation for the peer-tutoring phase displayed in Figure 16.

PREPARING CBM-TYPE GRAPHS

The use of CBM requires that specific types of graphs be generated. These graphs provide opportunities to collect data across a long period of time (usually an entire school year), and to incorporate goal setting and graphing of expected performance. For example, Dan is a beginning third-grade student. Baseline data taken over 3 days show that Dan is reading at 48 words correct per minute (WCPM), 30 WCPM, and 53 WCPM in third-grade material. Using scores collected during a

FIGURE 18. Illustration of the ordinary least squares (OLS) method of trend estimation for the peer-tutoring displayed in Figure 17D.

local norming project of Dan's school district, the teacher elects to set a yearly goal for Dan to read at the 50th percentile of third-grade readers by the end of the year—that is, a goal of 90 WCPM. Figure 19 shows the CBM graph generated. In the figure, Dan's baseline is represented by the median score across the three baseline data sessions (48 WCPM). A goal of 90 WCPM at the end of a 36-week period (one academic year from the time the data collection is started in September) is indicated on the graph, and a solid line connecting the baseline and goal is drawn. This line represents Dan's "aim line." As data are collected over time, it is anticipated that Dan's performance will match this line of progress. If his scores consistently exceed the aim line, then the teacher may decide to increase the goal originally set for Dan. If his scores consistently are below the aim line or move in a direction opposite to that shown by the aim line, the teacher should decide to alter the instructional technique to improve Dan's performance. Also, with the goal of 90 WCPM, Dan is expected to improve his oral reading fluency by 1.2 WCPM each week; this is his slope of expected improvement (90 WCPM – 48 WCPM = 42 WCPM ÷ 36 weeks = 1.2 WCPM/week).

Exercise 11 provides an opportunity to practice developing a CBM graph.

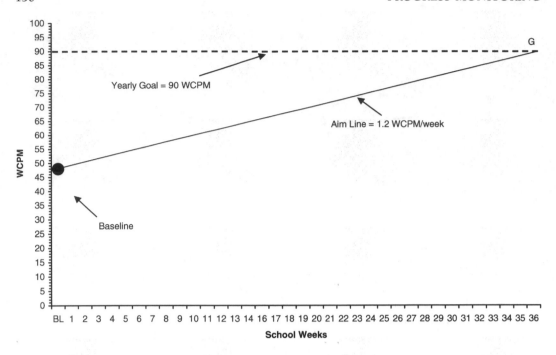

FIGURE 19. CBM graph showing Dan's baseline performance and expected rate of progress in reading across a school year.

DEVELOPING A CBM GRAPH

STUDENT

Betsy is a beginning fourth-grader. Her reading fluency at baseline is determined to be 40 WCPM in fourth-grade material, where she will be taught this year. Her teacher, looking to set a goal that placed her at least at the 25th percentile for fourth graders at the end of the year, selects 88 WCPM as her year-end goal. Biweekly monitoring of her reading performance is planned across the 36 weeks of the school year.

DATA

During the first 5 weeks of school, the teacher obtains the following data:

Week 1:	45 WCPM
	35 WCPM
Week 2:	50 WCPM
	46 WCPM
Week 3:	50 WCPM
	44 WCPM
Week 4:	48 WCPM
	56 WCPM
Week 5:	52 WCPM
	55 WCPM

INSTRUCTIONS

1. Construct a graph including an aim line.
2. Plot Betsy's actual performance.
3. Use the quarter intersect method to plot a trend estimation for Betsy's performance.
4. What might be the teacher's decision based on these data?

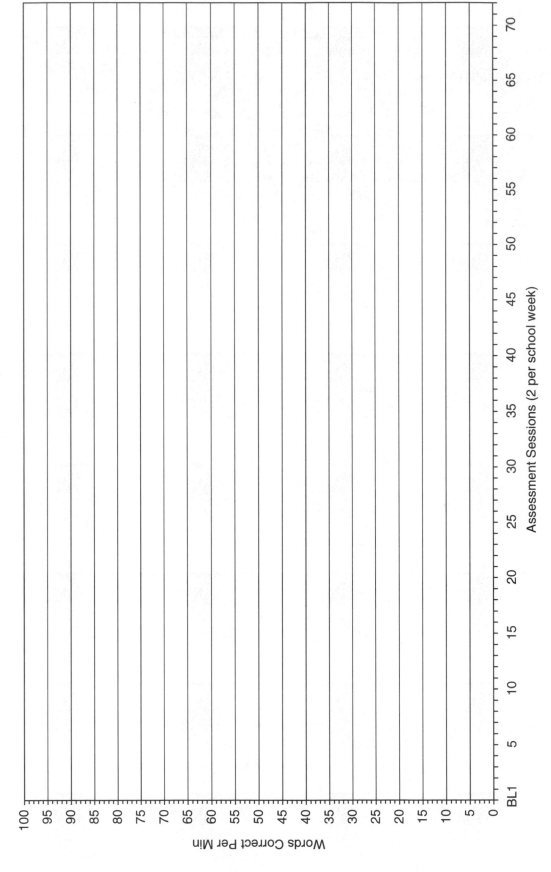

Progress Monitoring Graph in Reading for Betsy

Words Correct Per Min

Assessment Sessions (2 per school week)

132

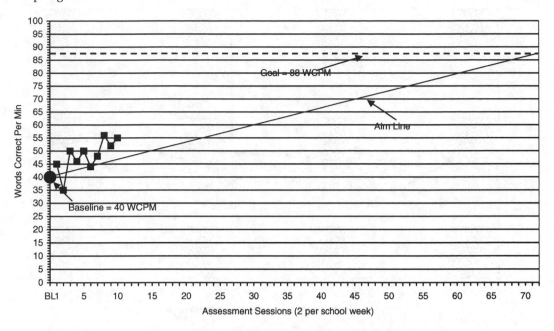

FIGURE 20. Progress monitoring graph for Betsy.

ANSWER FOR EXERCISE 11

The results of graphing Betsy's performance is shown in Figure 20. Trend lines using the quarter-intersect and the OLS methods are shown in Figure 21. In Betsy's case, both methods were approximately equal in showing her progress. Looking at Figure 22, the data show that Betsy is making greater progress than would be expected. As such, it is possible that the goal set for her is currently too low. The teacher may decide to reset the goal for Betsy at 98 rather than 88 WCPM. When the new goal line is drawn, a dashed vertical line is drawn on the graph, and the new aim line using a goal of 98 WCPM from the starting point (the baseline of 40 WCPM) is drawn between the dashed vertical line and the goal. Figure 23 shows the resulting CBM graph with the increased goal.

FIGURE 21. Quarter-intersect and OLS trend estimation for Betsy's reading progress.

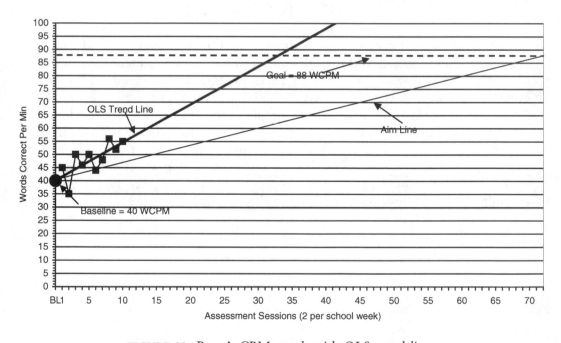

FIGURE 22. Betsy's CBM graph with OLS trend line.

FIGURE 23. CBM graph for Betsy, with goal raised from 88 to 98 WCPM.

♦♦♦
Developing Local Norms
♦

The process of selecting goals in CBA can be greatly enhanced by the use of local norms. Shinn (1988, 1989) provides an excellent discussion of this process and offers step-by-step directions on how to construct these norms. Specifically, Shinn (1988) notes that one must create a measurement net that defines the appropriate skills and materials for assessment, establish a normative sampling plan, train data collectors, have the data collected, and summarize the data. Gathering data that represent the performance of students within the schools where the data will be used provides a strong sense of the ownership of the outcomes, and increases the certainty that the data comparison will be representative of the community.

To illustrate this process, the steps involved in the collection of local norms in reading for elementary school students from a medium-size, urban school district are described. The reader should note that the sampling procedures used here are different than those recommended by Shinn (1988). The normative data from three districts are also presented, each representing high, moderate, and low levels of socioeconomic status, as defined by the percentage of low-income families in the district.

CREATING THE MEASUREMENT NET

The school district was using a literature-based reading program and wanted to use its own reading series to conduct the norms. Data were to be collected three times during the year: fall (October), winter (February), and spring (May). Reading levels of average students within grades were inconsistent across the district. At some schools, students were reading at levels commensurate with the publisher's assess-

TABLE 3. Measurement Net in Reading for Norming

Grade	Name of book	Publisher's assigned grade level
1	*Surprise*	1.4[a]
2	*Friends*	2.1[b]
3	*Just Listen*	3.1[b]
4	*Dinosauring*	4
5	*Explore*	5

[a]Indicates fourth book of grade level.
[b]Indicates first book of grade level.

ment of grade level of the material; in other schools, the majority of students were reading approximately one level (or book) behind. When this discrepancy was discussed, the school district decided to use the publisher-recommended grade-level material as the measures to be assessed. Passages for assessment were taken from materials that constituted the end-of-year goals for students in each grade, and each passage selected was evaluated using the Spache readability formula. Only passages that had readability levels within the grade-level book from which the passage was taken were used (see Table 3).

Randomly selected passages of between 150 and 200 words were selected from each book, according to standard CBM procedures. Passages were retyped on separate pages for presentation.

SELECTING THE SAMPLE

Given the size of the school district and resources available for data collection, it was not possible simply to select students randomly from across the district, as is often recommended in the process of obtaining local norms. In addition, the school district included a wide range of socioeconomic and academic ability levels that needed to be equally represented in the sample.

To address the problems of the resources available to collect the data, it was decided to concentrate the normative sample on six elementary schools. In considering the wide range of socioeconomic levels, the school district administrators identified six schools, two each that represented lower (L), lower middle (LM), and middle (M) socioeconomic levels (the three levels characterizing the district). To validate the selection of these schools, the percentages of students on free or reduced-fee lunches in the three schools were compared. The L schools identified had 93% of the students on free or reduced-fee lunches; the LM schools had 56%; and the M schools had 23%. Thus, these schools appeared to accurately represent the range of socioeconomic levels of the district.

The next problem was to develop a sample that would fairly represent the range of reading abilities within each of these schools. To accomplish this, prior to each scheduled assessment, the reading specialist assigned to each school provided a list of the current placement within the reading series of all students in that building. These data were used to identify the proportion of students in each grade within a building at each level of the reading series. For example, in the L schools, it was found that in the third grade, 10% of the students were reading in *Dinosauring* (fourth-grade book), 30% were reading in *Just Listen* (first book of third grade), 50% were reading in *Friends* (first book of the second grade), 8% were reading in *Surprises* (fourth book of the first grade), and 2% were reading below the first-grade level.

A normative sample consisting of a total of 900 students was developed, representing approximately 25% of the population of the three schools. From each school, 150 students (30 per grade) were selected. The normative sample within each school was constructed by selecting the identical proportion of students from each level of the reading series within each grade within each school. For example, to select the students from the third grade in the L school, the list of students placed in the *Just Listen* book was obtained. As noted earlier, this represented 30% of the third-grade students. Given that the final sample from the third grade of the L schools would have 30 students, a total of 4 (15% of 30) would be selected at random from among the possible 15% for inclusion in the normative sample. This process was repeated for each grade level and each school, in order to end up with a final sample whose representation was proportional to the percentage of students at the various reading levels of the grade.

DATA COLLECTION

Data were collected over 2-week periods in October, February, and May during the 1998–1999 school year. Graduate students in school psychology and special education served as data collectors. Students were tested on an individual basis in a small room adjacent to the classrooms in each of the school buildings. Each student was asked to read a passage aloud and was timed for 1 minute. The number of words read correct per minute was calculated according to standard CBM techniques. Errors included mispronunciations, omissions, and substitutions.

DATA ANALYSIS AND RESULTS

Results obtained from the normative data collection can be displayed in numerous ways. Table 4 and Figure 24 show the overall outcomes for the entire district. Such data as these can be used as the benchmarks for district's expectations and performance.

The data can also be broken down by individual schools. Figure 25 shows the 50th percentile performance levels across the six schools for the spring assessment. Examination of these data show that average student performances across the schools within the district were quite different. For example, in the third grade, it was found that the mean performance of students ranged from 40 in one L school to 115 in one of the M schools, a difference of 75 WCPM across these two schools. After third grade, these differences lessened, with the largest difference being 29 WCPM in the fifth grade across schools. Still, the data show that throughout all

TABLE 4. Quartiles for Local Norms in Reading from Grade-Level Reading
Material for a Medium-Size, Urban District in the Northeastern United States

Grade	Percentile	Fall	Winter	Spring
1	25th	1	2	6
	50th	2	5	13
	75th	6	15	35
2	25th	11	21	31
	50th	26	38	53
	75th	38	74	85
3	25th	36	38	44
	50th	50	63	78
	75th	81	95	118
4	25th	53	59	75
	50th	73	81	92
	75th	98	110	120
5	25th	77	83	88
	50th	98	110	121
	75th	130	142	151

grades and assessments across the school year, reading performance was clearly dif-
ferentiated by the school a student attended. Thus, a student reading at the 50th
percentile of the L school was often near or even below the 25th percentile of the M
school. Such data may be useful in helping teachers within schools predict expected
levels of performance; they may also assist administrators in setting schoolwide
goals for reading performance.

An important concern in using local norms is a recognition that a district's
overall level of academic performance is likely to vary very much based on the overall socioeconomic base of the district. Table 5 provides data from three districts
where local norms were collected. One of the districts has a high number of low-
income families (59.5%), the second a moderate level of low-income families
(32.8%), and the third a small number of low income families (6.3%). As can be
seen in Table 5, reading performance varied greatly across these districts. For example, students assessed in the spring of the third grade, who scored at the 25th percentile, ranged from 44 WCPM in the low-income district, 89 WCPM in the moderate-income district, and 102 WCPM in the high-income district. Although the
differences lessened as students reached the fifth-grade level, there was still a difference of 33 WCPM between the low- and high-income districts. Clearly, using local
norms places students' performance within the context of the environment in which
they are living. Using data such as those in Table 5 can allow a district to set ambi-
tious goals that may challenge students to reach levels of performance similar to
those districts that may have high-percentages of high-achieving students.

Although the example presented here used reading material that was from the
district's curriculum of instruction, it is neither required nor recommended that districts develop their own passages for norming purposes. Standard reading passages
that are closely controlled for grade-based readability are available from both commercial and free sites. Readers may want to examine these sources for reading pas-

FIGURE 24. Normative data in reading from midsize urban school district showing 25th and 75th percentiles across grades and assessment periods.

sages that have been found to be effective in conducting local norms in reading. Such passages are available commercially from several sources, such as AIMSweb (*http://www.aimsweb.com*), Scholastic Fluency (*http://teacher.scholastic. com*), Children's Educational Services (*http://www.readingprogress.com*), and Read Naturally (*http://readnaturally.com*). Materials for assessing prereading skills of emerging readers that include oral reading fluency passages up through sixth grade are also available (DIBELS: *http://dibels.uoregon.edu*).

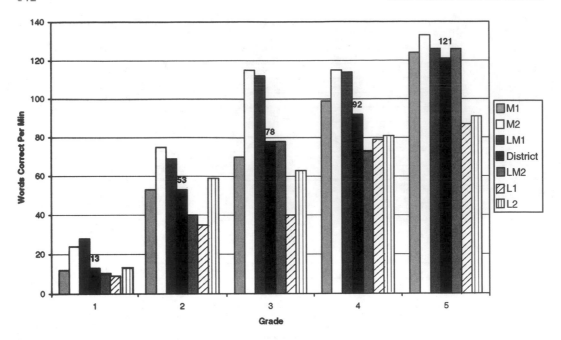

FIGURE 25. Comparisons of the 50th percentile at spring of six schools from a lower SES school district. The black bar represents the district mean. M, moderate-income school; LM, low–moderate-income school; L, low-income school.

TABLE 5. Words Correct per Minute Scores at the 25th Percentile across Three School Districts from High, Moderate, and Low Socioeconomic Bases

	Fall	Winter	Spring
Grade 1			
High	4	29	59
Moderate	4	15	26
Low	1	2	6
Grade 2			
High	31	69	79
Moderate	31	55	67
Low	11	21	31
Grade 3			
High	68	86	102
Moderate	62	77	89
Low	36	38	44
Grade 4			
High	80	98	114
Moderate	83	96	104
Low	53	59	75
Grade 5			
High	103	113	121
Moderate	90	101	115
Low	77	83	88

◆ ◆ ◆

Using Goal Charts

◆

Once local norms have been developed, evaluators can use these data both to establish a student's current level of performance and set a goal for expected performance. A tool that assists in goal setting is the use of goal charts. A goal chart plots the average student performance from the 25th to the 75th percentile for each grade. Using the chart, the performance of the student assessed is plotted on the chart. The outcome shows the contrast between the target student's reading level and the expected reading level for each student across each grade in which the student was assessed. Figure 26 shows an example of a goal chart for a student based on the winter assessment. The student, a third grader, was first tested in third-grade materials, where he was found to be reading at 33 WCPM. This was substantially below the 25th percentile for same-grade peers who were reading 77 WCPM. When tested in second-grade materials, he was found to be reading 35 WCPM, again, still below the 25th percentile of other second peers. In first-grade material, he was found to be reading at 50 WCPM, which was well within the 25th to 75th percentile band of comparison for first-grade students in his district.

Based on the analysis of his data, the decision is made that although his performance is just below the instructional level (25th percentile) at second grade, that would be the appropriate level of material in which he should be taught. First-grade material is well within his instructional level and, therefore, probably does not present enough challenge for him.

To set a reasonable goal using the goal chart, the evaluator would examine what level the student would need to reach by the end of the school year (spring) to reach at least the 25th percentile of performance. As seen in Table 5, the student would need to reach 89 WCPM to achieve reading comparable to peers for the district in third-grade material. Thus, the student would need to increase from 35

FIGURE 26. Goal chart for reading for a third grader in a high-SES school district.

WCPM in second-grade material to 89 WCPM in third-grade material, a gain of 54 WCPM across the final 18 weeks of school, or 3.0 WCPM per week. When the teacher considered this level of gain, she decided that such an improvement would be much too challenging for the student. Instead, she examined what the 25th percentile for second-grade students would be in second-grade material by the end of the year. Examining the goal chart for second-grade students at the end of the year (Figure 27), she finds that 67 WCPM in second-grade material would equal levels of other students in the district who are reading at the 25th percentile. Because she wants her student to achieve better than the 25th percentile, she chooses 76 WCPM as the target goal. This would be a gain of 41 WCPM across 18 weeks of school in second-grade material, or a gain of 2.3 WCPM per week in second-grade material. The teacher believes this to be a challenging yet realistic goal, and establishes a CBM chart to monitor the student's progress twice per week in reading with the aim line set at 2.3 WCPM.

Goal charts, such as those shown in Figures 26 and 27 can be easily developed using graphing and spreadsheet programs such as Microsoft EXCEL, Quatro-Pro, or Delta Graph.

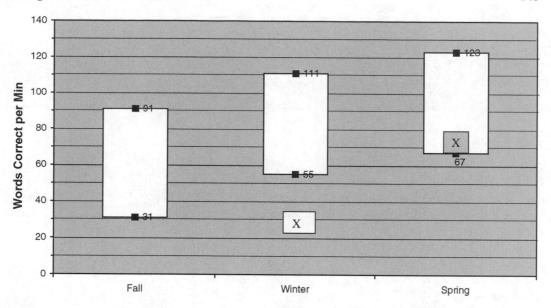

FIGURE 27. Goal chart for reading for second-grade students in a high-SES school district.

◆◆◆
References
◆

Burns, M. K. (2001). Measuring sight-word acquisition and retention rates with curriculum-based assessment. *Journal of Psychoeducational Assessment, 19,* 148–157.

DuPaul, G. J., Rapport, M. D., & Perriello, L. M. (1991). Teacher ratings of academic skills: The development of the Academic Performance Rating Scale. *School Psychology Review, 20,* 284–300.

Fuchs, L. S., & Fuchs, D. (1992). Identifying a measure for monitoring student reading progress. *School Psychology Review, 21,* 45–58.

Fuchs, L. S., Fuchs, D., Hamlett, C. L., & Allinder, R. M. (1991). Effects of expert system advice within curriculum-based measurement on teacher planning and student achievement in spelling. *School Psychology Review, 20,* 49–66.

Fuchs, L. S., Hamlett, C. L., & Fuchs, D. (1990). *Monitoring basic skills progress: Basic spelling.* Austin, TX: Pro-Ed.

Fuchs, L. S., Hamlett, C. L., & Fuchs, D. (1999a). *Monitoring basic skills progress: Basic math concepts and applications* [computer program]. Austin, TX: Pro-Ed.

Fuchs, L. S., Hamlett, C. L., & Fuchs, D. (1999b). *Monitoring basic skills progress: Basic reading* (2nd ed) [computer program]. Austin, TX: Pro-Ed.

Gickling, E. E., & Havertape, S. (1981). *Curriculum-based assessment (CBA).* Minneapolis, MN: School Psychology Inservice Training Network.

Hargis, C. H., Terhaar-Yonker, M., Williams, P. C., & Reed, M. T. (1988). Repetition requirements for word recognition. *Journal of Reading, 31,* 320–327.

MacQuarrie, L. L., Tucker, J. A., Burns, M. L., & Hartman, B. (2002). Comparison of retention rates using traditional, drill sandwich, and incremental rehearsal flash card methods. *School Psychology Review, 31,* 584–595.

Shapiro, E. S. (2004). *Academic skills problems: Direct assessment and intervention* (3rd ed.). New York: Guilford Press.

Shinn, M. R. (1988). Development of curriculum-based local norms for use in special education decision-making. *School Psychology Review, 17,* 61–80.

Shinn, M. R. (1989). *Curriculum-based measurement: Assessing special children.* New York: Guilford Press.

White, O. R., & Haring, N. G. (1980). *Exceptional teaching* (2nd ed.). Columbus, OH: Merrill.